SpringerBriefs in Modern Perspectives on Disability Research

This book series on disability research is a comprehensive collection of research on disability and related issues. The series is designed to promote interdisciplinary collaboration and exchange, bringing together scholars and practitioners from different fields to share their perspectives and insights. Disability research is an interdisciplinary field that examines the social, cultural, historical, and political dimensions of disability. It encompasses a wide range of topics, including disability rights, accessibility, assistive technologies, healthcare, education, employment, and social welfare. Disability research scholars employ a range of theoretical and methodological approaches to understand the experiences of people with disabilities, as well as the ways in which disability intersects with other social identities such as race, gender, sexuality, and class.

The series seeks to advance knowledge and understanding of disability by publishing rigorous, innovative, and relevant research. It aims to promote disability rights and social justice by highlighting the ways in which people with disabilities are marginalized and discriminated against in society, and advocating for greater social inclusion and accessibility. The series also seeks to inform policy and practice by disseminating research findings that can help to shape policy decisions and contribute to positive social change.

Mohammad Hossein Rouhani • Fatemeh Navab •
Farnaz Shahdadian • Shayesteh Keyhanpour

The Healing Plate

Nutritional Strategies for Common Disability Disorders

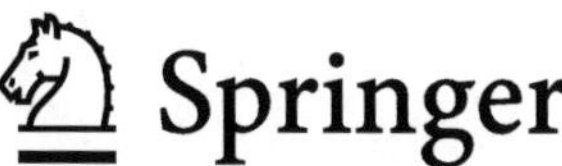

Mohammad Hossein Rouhani
Nutrition and Food Security Research Center and Department of Clinical Nutrition, School of Nutrition and Food Science
Isfahan University of Medical Sciences
Isfahan, Iran

Fatemeh Navab
Nutrition and Food Security Research Center and Department of Clinical Nutrition, School of Nutrition and Food Science
Isfahan University of Medical Sciences
Isfahan, Iran

Farnaz Shahdadian
Nutrition and Food Security Research Center and Department of Clinical Nutrition, School of Nutrition and Food Science
Isfahan University of Medical Sciences
Isfahan, Iran

Shayesteh Keyhanpour
Nutrition and Food Security Research Center and Department of Clinical Nutrition, School of Nutrition and Food Science
Isfahan University of Medical Sciences
Isfahan, Iran

ISSN 3004-9709 ISSN 3004-9717 (electronic)
SpringerBriefs in Modern Perspectives on Disability Research
ISBN 978-981-95-8149-8 ISBN 978-981-95-8150-4 (eBook)
https://doi.org/10.1007/978-981-95-8150-4

This Springer imprint is published by the registered company Springer Nature Singapore Pte Ltd.
The registered company address is: 152 Beach Road, #21-01/04 Gateway East, Singapore 189721, Singapore

Dedication
To my family and friends, for their encouragement and support.

Preface

This book is the outcome of several research efforts on the importance of nutrition in the prevention and management of disability disorders. Our aim was to summarize the essential concepts that dietitians can apply in practice, without focusing extensively on biological pathways or molecular mechanisms.

The book is intended for dietitians as well as undergraduate and postgraduate students of nutrition.

I would like to thank Springer for providing my colleagues and me with the opportunity to prepare this book. My heartfelt gratitude also goes to my co-authors, whose dedication and diligence made this work possible.

Isfahan, Iran

Mohammad Hossein Rouhani
Fatemeh Navab
Farnaz Shahdadian
Shayesteh Keyhanpour

Acknowledgments

This book could not have been prepared without the heartfelt contributions and encouragement of my colleagues at School of Nutrition and Food Science, Isfahan University of Medical Sciences. I would like to express my sincere gratitude to my students, who played a key role in conducting the research projects.

Finally, I extend my deepest and most sincere thanks to my family, whose support and encouragement have been my primary motivation throughout this work.

Competing Interests The authors have no competing interests to declare that are relevant to the content of this manuscript.

About the Book

This book highlights the crucial role of dietary intake in the prevention and management of disability disorders. It provides an overview of the most prevalent nutrition-related conditions, including Down syndrome, autism, cerebral palsy, attention-deficit/hyperactivity disorder, stress, anxiety, depression, Alzheimer's disease, schizophrenia, Parkinson's disease, stroke, multiple sclerosis, and Guillain-Barré syndrome. Designed as a concise yet comprehensive guide, it serves dietitians, nutritionists, and healthcare professionals seeking practical insights. In addition, the book addresses nutritional challenges and food–drug interactions, making it a valuable resource for both clinical practice and academic study.

Contents

About the Authors

Mohammad Hossein Rouhani is a researcher and academic specializing in nutrition and its role in disability and neurodevelopmental disorders. His scholarly work has been published in high-impact journals. He has investigated the associations between dietary patterns, dietary acid load, polyphenol intake, inflammatory indices, and mental health outcomes, with a particular focus on attention-deficit/hyperactivity disorder (ADHD) and related conditions. Dr. Rouhani's research highlights the importance of nutritional strategies in both prevention and management of disability-related disorders, providing evidence-based insights into how dietary factors influence neurological, psychological, and physical health. Beyond his academic contributions, he has been actively engaged in clinical nutrition practice and the development of dietary guidelines, aiming to translate scientific findings into practical recommendations for healthcare professionals.

Fatemeh Navab is a researcher and academic specializing in clinical nutrition and its applications in chronic diseases. As a PhD candidate in Nutritional Sciences at Isfahan University of Medical Sciences, she has authored multiple peer-reviewed publications in high-impact journals and contributed to several specialized books in therapeutic nutrition.

Her scholarly work has explored the complex interplay between dietary patterns, micronutrient status, and neurological outcomes, with a particular emphasis on attention-deficit/hyperactivity disorder (ADHD) and related disabling conditions.

Beyond her academic publications, Navab is a co-inventor of a registered patent in functional food innovation. She has also served as a speaker at national and international congresses, actively working to bridge the gap between evidence-based research and clinical nutrition practice.

Farnaz Shahdadian is a researcher and academic specializing in the intersection of dietary patterns, mental health, and disability disorders. Her research emphasizes the role of dietary quality and patterns in modulating stress, emotional regulation, and mood disorders, as well as the impact of the gut–brain axis and metabolic pathways on mental health. In addition, Dr. Shahdadian investigates nutritional and lifestyle interventions designed to support individuals living with neurodevelopmental or acquired disabilities, aiming to enhance quality of life and functional outcomes.

She has contributed to peer-reviewed publications, presented findings at national and international scientific meetings, and collaborated with interdisciplinary teams working at the intersection of neuro-nutrition, psychology, and public health. Through this work, Dr. Shahdadian seeks to bridge the gap between epidemiological evidence and clinical application, highlighting the potential of evidence-based dietary strategies as complementary tools in the management of psychological disorders and disability-related conditions.

Chapter 1
Introduction

1.1 Background

Disability disorders (DDs) encompass a wide range of diseases and syndromes that pose a major global health challenge and profoundly affect both personal and social life. Individuals with DDs often experience reduced quality of life, high healthcare costs, diminished self-confidence, poor social participation, and limited work capacity. Furthermore, the presence of a family member with a disability negatively impacts the overall well-being of the household, as other members are required to devote time to caregiving and redirect financial resources toward healthcare expenses rather than quality-of-life improvements.

According to the World Health Organization, approximately 1.3 billion people worldwide live with some form of disability—equivalent to 16% of the global population, or one in six individuals (World Health Organization, n.d.-a). Data from European countries show a 25% increase in the prevalence of disability over the past decade, with the sharpest rise observed in individuals aged 85 years and older (Guzman-Castillo et al., 2017). Similarly, data from the CDC's Disability and Health Data System indicate that nearly 30% of U.S. adults report a functional disability, including impairments in hearing, vision, mobility, cognition, self-care, or independent living (Centers for Disease Control and Prevention, 2025). The South-East Asia Region is recognized as one of the most affected areas globally, with over 15% of the population experiencing disability, a considerable proportion of whom suffer from severe forms (World Health Organization, n.d.-b). With global aging trends, the prevalence of DDs is expected to rise substantially in the coming decades.

Disability disorders encompass diverse conditions, which may be classified into five main categories:

1. Mobility and physical capacity disorders—such as multiple sclerosis, Guillain-Barré syndrome, and cerebral palsy.

M. H. Rouhani et al., *The Healing Plate*, SpringerBriefs in Modern Perspectives on Disability Research, https://doi.org/10.1007/978-981-95-8150-4_1

2. Acquired brain injuries, including stroke-related disability, which occur after birth and result in functional impairment.
3. Neurological disabilities—involving damage to the nervous system, such as Parkinson's disease and Alzheimer's disease.
4. Neurodevelopmental disorders, including autism spectrum disorder (ASD), Down syndrome, and attention-deficit/hyperactivity disorder (ADHD).
5. Psychiatric disabilities, where mental health conditions such as schizophrenia, stress-related disorders, anxiety, and depression lead to significant functional impairments.

1.2 Diet and Disability Disorders

Given this heterogeneity, the etiology of DDs is highly diverse and shaped by multiple environmental and socioeconomic factors. Socioeconomic status (SES) is particularly influential. Higher education levels are associated with a reduced risk of developing functional disability later in life (Nurrika et al., 2019), while greater income provides better access to healthcare services (Qiu et al., 2023). Epidemiological evidence indicates that conditions such as epilepsy, cerebral palsy, and ASD are more prevalent and severe in populations with low SES. Contributing factors include pregnancy complications, poor maternal nutrition, limited healthcare access, and greater exposure to environmental toxins.

Among environmental influences, dietary intake plays a crucial role in both the prevention and management of DDs. A growing body of evidence supports the impact of specific dietary patterns on the risk and progression of these disorders (Kilpinen-Loisa et al., 2009; Park et al., 2012).

The Gluten-Free/Casein-Free (GFCF) diet involves eliminating gluten-containing grains (wheat, rye, barley, and oats) and casein from dairy products (cow, goat, and sheep). Gluten-free substitutes are typically used, and in some cases both restrictions are combined to minimize dietary triggers (Reissmann, 2020; Zafirovski et al., 2024). A systematic review and meta-analysis reported beneficial effects of GFCF on behavior, language, and social interaction in children with DDs (Karimi et al., 2024).

The Ketogenic Diet (KD), characterized by low carbohydrate and high fat intake, induces hepatic production of ketone bodies (acetoacetate, β-hydroxybutyrate, and acetone), thereby shifting the body's primary energy source from glucose to ketones.

KD has been linked to improved metabolic regulation, effective seizure control, and potential benefits for cognitive development and social functioning (Dyńka et al., 2022; Li et al., 2021; McGaugh & Barthel, 2022).

The Specific Carbohydrate Diet (SCD) restricts simple carbohydrates and limits complex carbohydrates to improve nutrient absorption. It has been proposed to support intestinal healing, limit pathogenic bacterial growth, and restore gut microbiota balance. SCD has shown therapeutic promise for irritable bowel syndrome, celiac disease, and ASD. The diet prioritizes fermented foods (e.g., homemade yogurt, probiotic products), alongside meat, poultry, fish, eggs, fruits, vegetables, nuts, and seeds, while excluding starches. Typically, it begins with a limited food list that gradually expands as gastrointestinal function improves (Ābele et al., 2021; Hagström et al., 2025; Obih et al., 2016).

The Body Ecology Diet (BED) was developed to reduce Candida albicans overgrowth, improve gut health, and maintain acid–base balance. It emphasizes low-acid, easily digestible foods and includes a wide range of fermented products such as sauerkraut, kefir, and plant-based yogurts. Naturally gluten-free, BED excludes rice, corn, and soy but allows properly prepared grains such as quinoa, millet, amaranth, and whole wheat. Its relevance in ASD stems from evidence linking Candida overgrowth with behavioral disturbances (e.g., aggression, hyperactivity, poor attention) and somatic symptoms such as headaches, gastrointestinal discomfort, fatigue, and depression. In practice, BED is often combined with antifungal therapy and probiotic supplementation (Gates & Schatz, 2011).

The Elimination Diet targets food sensitivities by removing common allergens such as eggs, milk, wheat, soy, peanuts, tree nuts, and fish/shellfish. In severe cases, the diet is restricted to hypoallergenic foods only. This approach is mainly used to identify and manage food intolerances that may exacerbate gastrointestinal or behavioral symptoms in autism (Krishnamurthy et al., 2024; Ly et al., 2017).

The Additive- and Food Dye-Free Diet removes synthetic colorants (Blue 1 and 2, Citrus Red 2, Green 3, Red 40, Yellow 5 and 6) and preservatives such as sodium benzoate. The strategy is designed to limit artificial additives that may contribute to behavioral or gastrointestinal disturbances, particularly in children with ASD (Karaca Şahin et al., 2025; Sultana et al., 2023; Wender, 1986).

1.3 Malnutrition and Disability Disorders

Nutrition plays a fundamental role in health promotion and disease prevention, and research consistently shows that a healthy diet improves both quality and length of life. For individuals with primary disabilities, nutrition is critical, as they frequently face "secondary conditions," including additional medical, psychological, or functional problems that may worsen their overall health and limit participation in daily activities. Unlike the primary disability, these secondary conditions are considered preventable or modifiable through appropriate interventions, with nutrition serving as both a risk factor and a protective factor (Holden & Corby, 2019; Humphries et al., 2002; Koritsas & Iacono, 2011).

The relationship between malnutrition and disability is bidirectional. Malnutrition, whether due to macronutrient or micronutrient deficiencies, can contribute to the development of physical, sensory, and cognitive impairments across the lifespan. During fetal development, maternal undernutrition, including deficiencies in folate, vitamin D, and calcium, increases the risk of serious disability disorders. Folate insufficiency is strongly linked to neural tube defects, while inadequate vitamin D or calcium during pregnancy raises the likelihood of preterm birth, a condition associated with multiple complications and long-term outcomes such as cerebral palsy, as well as cognitive, visual, and hearing impairments. In infancy and early childhood, underweight and stunting further elevate the risk of developmental delays. Conversely, many disabilities increase vulnerability to malnutrition, as seen in cerebral palsy, craniofacial anomalies, and genetic syndromes such as Down syndrome, where feeding and swallowing difficulties, nutrient malabsorption, and higher energy demands are common (AbdAllah et al., 2007; Blencowe et al., 2010; Gottlieb et al., 2009; Groce et al., 2013; Groce et al., 2014; Kerac et al., 2014; Maulik & Darmstadt, 2007; Tüzün et al., 2013; Wagner & Brath, 2012).

Malnutrition in persons with disabilities is associated with higher morbidity and mortality, delayed recovery, poorer developmental outcomes, and in severe cases, death. Addressing these challenges requires individualized medical nutrition therapy, training of caregivers and health professionals in basic nutrition and food safety, and ongoing follow-up to prevent the vicious cycle of disability, malnutrition, and declining health (Groce et al., 2014; Kerac et al., 2014; Werner, 1987).

1.4 Aims

Given the critical role of nutrition in management of disability disorders, preventing complications, improving functional outcomes, and enhancing quality of life across these five domains of disability, the following chapters of this book will explore nutritional management in detail. These chapters aim to provide evidence-based guidance for healthcare providers and caregivers, emphasizing practical strategies to optimize growth, maintain functional capacity, and manage nutrition-related secondary conditions such as malnutrition, obesity, and micronutrient deficiencies. The ultimate goal is to empower individuals with disability disorders to achieve better health and well-being through tailored and scientifically grounded nutritional care.

Acknowledgments The authors confirm that the content, analysis, and conclusions of this manuscript are their own work. AI-based tools were used solely to assist in improving the clarity and correctness of the English language.

References

AbdAllah, A. M., El-Sherbeny, S. S., & Khairy, S. (2007). Nutritional status of mentally disabled children in Egypt. *The Egyptian Journal of Hospital Medicine, 29*(1), 604–615.

Ābele, S., Meija, L., Folkmanis, V., & Tzivian, L. (2021). Specific carbohydrate diet (SCD/GAPS) and dietary supplements for children with autistic spectrum disorder. *Proceedings of the Latvian Academy of Sciences, 75*, 417. De Gruyter Poland.

Blencowe, H., Cousens, S., Modell, B., & Lawn, J. (2010). Folic acid to reduce neonatal mortality from neural tube disorders. *International Journal of Epidemiology, 39*(suppl_1), i110–ii21.

Centers for Disease Control and Prevention. (2025). *Disability and health data now: CDC / centers for disease control and prevention*. Retrieved April 8, 2025, from https://www.cdc.gov/disability-and-health/articles-documents

Dyńka, D., Kowalcze, K., & Paziewska, A. (2022). The role of ketogenic diet in the treatment of neurological diseases. *Nutrients, 14*(23), 5003.

Gates, D., & Schatz, L. (2011). *The body ecology diet: Recovering your health and rebuilding your immunity*. Hay House.

Gottlieb, C. A., Maenner, M. J., Cappa, C., & Durkin, M. S. (2009). Child disability screening, nutrition, and early learning in 18 countries with low and middle incomes: Data from the third round of UNICEF's multiple indicator cluster survey (2005–06). *The Lancet, 374*(9704), 1831–1839.

Groce, N., Challenger, E., Berman-Bieler, R., Farkas, A., Yilmaz, N., Schultink, W., et al. (2014). Malnutrition and disability: Unexplored opportunities for collaboration. *Paediatrics and International Child Health, 34*(4), 308–314.

Groce, N. E., Kerac, M., Farkas, A., Schultink, W., & Bieler, R. B. (2013). Inclusive nutrition for children and adults with disabilities. *The Lancet Global Health, 1*(4), e180–e1e1.

Guzman-Castillo, M., Ahmadi-Abhari, S., Bandosz, P., Capewell, S., Steptoe, A., Singh-Manoux, A., et al. (2017). Forecasted trends in disability and life expectancy in England and Wales up to 2025: A modelling study. *The Lancet Public Health, 2*(7), e307–ee13.

Hagström, N., Koochek, A., Lemming, E. W., Öman, A., Arnell, H., & Berntson, L. (2025). Exploring nutritional risks of the specific carbohydrate diet: Food and nutrient intake in children with juvenile idiopathic arthritis. *Journal of Nutritional Science, 14*, e9.

Holden, J., & Corby, N. (2019). *Disability and nutrition programming: Evidence and learning*. UKAID.

Humphries, K., Traci, M., Seekins, Ph. D. T., & Brusin, J. (2002). *Nutrition and disability*.

Karaca Şahin, M., Karamanlı, G., Çakar, N. E., & Özçeker, D. (2025). Sensitivity to food additives in autism spectrum disorder: Effects and implications. *International Journal of Developmental Disabilities*, 1–6.

Karimi, P., Deldar, M., & Sayehmiri, K. (2024). The effects of a gluten-free/casein-free diet on behavioral indices in children with autism Spectrum disorder: A systematic review and meta-analysis. *Iranian Journal of Pediatrics, 34*, e140372.

Kerac, M., Bunn, J., Chagaluka, G., Bahwere, P., Tomkins, A., Collins, S., et al. (2014). Follow-up of post-discharge growth and mortality after treatment for severe acute malnutrition (FuSAM study): A prospective cohort study. *PLoS One, 9*(6), e96030.

Kerac, M., Postels, D. G., Mallewa, M., Jalloh, A. A., Voskuijl, W. P., Groce, N., et al. (2014). The interaction of malnutrition and neurologic disability in Africa. *Seminars in Pediatric Neurology, 21*, 42. Elsevier.

Kilpinen-Loisa, P., Pihko, H., Vesander, U., Paganus, A., Ritanen, U., & Mäkitie, O. (2009). Insufficient energy and nutrient intake in children with motor disability. *Acta Paediatrica, 98*(8), 1329–1333.

Koritsas, S., & Iacono, T. (2011). Secondary conditions in people with developmental disability. *American Journal of Intellectual and Developmental Disabilities, 116*(1), 36–47.

Krishnamurthy, H. K., Pereira, M., Jayaraman, V., Krishna, K., Wang, T., Bei, K., & et al. (2024). *Personalized food elimination diet: A clinical trial based on food sensitivity assessment*.

Li, Q., Liang, J., Fu, N., Han, Y., & Qin, J. (2021). A ketogenic diet and the treatment of autism spectrum disorder. *Frontiers in Pediatrics, 9*, 650624.

Ly, V., Bottelier, M., Hoekstra, P. J., Arias Vasquez, A., Buitelaar, J. K., & Rommelse, N. N. (2017). Elimination diets' efficacy and mechanisms in attention deficit hyperactivity disorder and autism spectrum disorder. *European Child & Adolescent Psychiatry, 26*(9), 1067–1079.

Maulik, P. K., & Darmstadt, G. L. (2007). Childhood disability in low-and middle-income countries: Overview of screening, prevention, services, legislation, and epidemiology. *Pediatrics, 120*(Supplement_1), S1–S55.

McGaugh, E., & Barthel, B. (2022). A review of ketogenic diet and lifestyle. *Missouri Medicine, 119*(1), 84.

Nurrika, D., Zhang, S., Tomata, Y., Sugawara, Y., Tanji, F., & Tsuji, I. (2019). Education level and incident functional disability in elderly Japanese: The Ohsaki Cohort 2006 study. *PLoS One, 14*(3), e0213386.

Obih, C., Wahbeh, G., Lee, D., Braly, K., Giefer, M., Shaffer, M. L., et al. (2016). Specific carbohydrate diet for pediatric inflammatory bowel disease in clinical practice within an academic IBD center. *Nutrition, 32*(4), 418–425.

Park, S., Cho, S.-C., Hong, Y.-C., Oh, S.-Y., Kim, J.-W., Shin, M.-S., et al. (2012). Association between dietary behaviors and attention-deficit/hyperactivity disorder and learning disabilities in school-aged children. *Psychiatry Research, 198*(3), 468–476.

Qiu, N., Jiang, Y., Sun, Z., & Du, M. (2023). The impact of disability-related deprivation on employment opportunity at the neighborhood level: Does family socioeconomic status matter? *Frontiers in Public Health, 11*, 1232829.

Reissmann, A. (2020). Gluten-free and casein-free diets in the management of autism spectrum disorder: A systematic literature review. *Movement and Nutrition in Health and Disease, 4*, 21.

Sultana, S., Rahman, M. M., Aovi, F. I., Jahan, F. I., Hossain, M. S., Brishti, S. A., et al. (2023). Food color additives in hazardous consequences of human health: An overview. *Current Topics in Medicinal Chemistry, 23*(14), 1380–1393.

Tüzün, E. H., Güven, D. K., Eker, L., Elbasan, B., & Bülbül, S. F. (2013). Nutritional status of children with cerebral palsy in Turkey. *Disability and Rehabilitation, 35*(5), 413–417.

Wagner, K.-H., & Brath, H. (2012). A global view on the development of non communicable diseases. *Preventive Medicine, 54*, S38–S41.

Wender, E. H. (1986). The food additive-free diet in the treatment of behavior disorders: A review. *Journal of Developmental and Behavioral Pediatrics, 7*(1), 35–42.

Werner, D. (1987). *Disabled village children*. The Hesperian Fdn.

World Health Organization. (n.d.-a). *Disability: WHO / world health organization*. https://www.who.int/health-topics/disability

World Health Organization. (n.d.-b). *Disability (South-East Asia): WHO / world health organization*. https://www.who.int/southeastasia/health-topics/disability

Zafirovski, K., Aleksoska, M. T., Thomas, J., & Hanna, F. (2024). Impact of gluten-free and casein-free diet on behavioural outcomes and quality of life of autistic children and adolescents: A scoping review. *Children, 11*(7), 862.

Chapter 2
Nutritional Assessment in Neurological Diseases

Abstract

- Nutritional assessment is a key step in managing neurological diseases, enabling identification of nutrition-related problems and guiding tailored interventions.
- Anthropometric evaluation includes height, weight, body mass index, and current-to-ideal weight ratio as basic indicators.
- Additional measurements such as triceps skin-fold thickness, mid-arm circumference, and mid-arm muscle circumference provide information on fat and muscle reserves.
- Bio-electrical impedance analysis offers non-invasive, rapid assessment of body composition, including fat, muscle, and water distribution.
- Biochemical and clinical assessments detect nutrient deficiencies and metabolic imbalances that may not be evident from dietary evaluation alone.
- Common biochemical markers include electrolytes, glucose, albumin, transthyretin, hemoglobin & hematocrit, cholesterol, triglycerides, vitamins B12, D, folate, trace elements (Fe, Zn, Cu), C-reactive protein, liver and kidney function tests, cerebrospinal fluid biomarkers, and selected genetic/metabolic tests.
- Clinical assessment evaluates developmental delays, sleep disturbances, mobility, neurological signs, autonomic dysfunction, and neuropsychiatric symptoms.
- Dietary intake is estimated using food diaries, 24-h recalls, or food frequency questionnaires; three to seven-day food diaries are most reliable.

Keywords Nutritional assessment · Disability disorders · Anthropometric measurements · Biochemical markers · Clinical evaluation · Dietary intake · Malnutrition · Body composition · Micronutrients

Nutritional assessment is an essential process in managing patients with disability disorders. It involves the systematic collection, evaluation, and interpretation of data to identify nutrition-related problems and formulate appropriate nutritional interventions. The nutritional assessment includes anthropometric measurements, biochemical tests, clinical evaluation, and dietary intake analysis, which together inform the development of a tailored nutritional care plan (Lee, 2022).

M. H. Rouhani et al., *The Healing Plate*, SpringerBriefs in Modern Perspectives on Disability Research, https://doi.org/10.1007/978-981-95-8150-4_2

2.1 Anthropometric Assessment

Anthropometric evaluation is a simple and economical method for assessing nutritional status. Basic parameters such as height, weight, body mass index (BMI), and the ratio of current to ideal or usual body weight are commonly used as initial indicators (Luft et al., 2008). In addition, triceps skin-fold thickness, mid-arm circumference, and mid-arm muscle circumference can provide estimates of fat and muscle reserves. Bio-electrical impedance analysis (BIA) is also a practical tool to assess body composition, offering a rapid and non-invasive evaluation of fat, muscle, and water distribution (Lee, 2022).

2.2 Biochemical and Clinical Assessment in Specific Disability Disorders

Biochemical and clinical indicators play a key role in evaluating both nutritional status and general health. They offer measurable information on nutrient concentrations, metabolic processes, and organ performance, enabling the detection of deficiencies or imbalances that may not be evident through dietary assessment by itself (Team FC, 2025). Table 2.1 presents the biochemical (de Gonzalo-Calvo et al., 2020; Dorszewska & Kozubski, 2016; Harale et al., 2024; Hurjui et al., 2025; Khandelwal et al., 2023; Nayak et al., 2011; Niedziela et al., 2018; Nikouei Moghaddam et al., 2021; Paneyala et al., 2024; Polat et al., 2021; Rabbito et al., 2020; S E-S., 2022; Salman et al., 2021; Salvatore Orefice et al., 2012; Senarathne et al., 2023; Team FC, 2025; Wang et al., 2024; Yahya et al., 2023) and clinical assessment in specific disability disorders (Aborageh et al., 2025; Aging NIo, 2022; Ahmed et al., 2022; Ahuja et al., 2013; Ballal et al., 2024; Berardelli et al., 2001; Binda et al., 2024; Christogianni et al., 2018; Cizza et al., 2010; Cooper et al., 2023; Costi et al., 2020; De Georgia et al., 2023; Deramore Denver et al., 2016; Dyck & Piek, 2014; Farmakidis et al., 2015; Fernando & Goldman, 2019; Ferrarelli, 2021; Fields et al., 2021; Fritz et al., 2020; Fu et al., 2025; Goffinski et al., 2015; Goodman et al., 2015; Gur et al., 2006; Horan et al., 2006; Huang et al., 2024; Hvolby, 2015; Jehan et al., 2018; Kahle et al., 2021; Kim et al., 2016; Koga et al., 2001; Köhler et al., 2016; Kwok & Schooling, 2021; Lan & Chen, 2012; Latif et al., 2024; Lee, 2021; Li et al., 2023; Malak et al., 2015; Mark & Duff, 2023; Marsh, 2013; Maure-Blesa et al., 2025; Meena et al., 2011; MHDSA, 2024; Nurković et al., 2020; Palakurthi & Burugupally, 2019; Parker & James, 1985; Ranjani et al., 2014; Roberts et al., 2019; Sand et al., 2012; Sarathy et al., 2019; Society NMS, 2025; Solaro et al., 2006; Solomon et al., 2008; Soryal et al., 1992; Stroke NIoNDa, 2025; Torsney et al., 2014; Waltz & Gold, 2015; Yeo et al., 2012).

Table 2.1 Biochemical and clinical assessment in specific disability disorders

Disease name	Biochemical assessment	Clinical assessment
Down syndrome	Ca^{2+}, Mg^{2+}, Na^{+}, K^{+}, Gluc, UA, Chol, LDL, trig, thyroid tests, folate, vitamin D, Zn, tHcy	Developmental delay, history of prematurity, OSA, Hyperextensibility of joints, large tongue
Autism Spectrum disorder	CBC with differential, Alb, TTR, Gluc, Chol, trig, celiac screening panel, lactose breath test, Fe^{2+}, ferritin, folate, glutathione (reduced), glutathione disulfide (oxidized), CRP, LFTs, thyroid tests, RAST / allergy testing, vitamin D, Zn, Lead (if pica behaviors present)	Endoscopy, pica, sleep patterns
Cerebral palsy	Alb, AlkP, Ca^{2+}, Mg^{2+}, Gluc, H&H, Fe^{2+}, ferritin, TFN	Activities scale for kids, DXA scan, functional mobility scale, gastroesophageal reflux disease, seizures / epilepsy, vision testing
Attention deficit hyperactivity disorder	Alb, TTR, Gluc, H&H, Fe^{2+}, ferritin, Chol, trig, LFTs, CK, vitamin D, Zn, cortisol, IL-6, TNF-α, Lead	Anxiety or depression, developmental delay, intellectual disability, irritability, epilepsy, sleep disturbances, pesticide exposure
Stress, anxiety, and major depressive disorder	Alb, TTR, H&H, Gluc Chol, trig, LFTs, Na^{+}, K^{+}, Ca^{2+}, Mg^{2+}, Fe^{2+}, ferritin, Cu^{2+}, Zn, CRP, thyroid tests, folate, vitamin B12, vitamin D, BUN, Creat, LDH, tHcy, serotonin, N balance, MTHFR mutation test	BP, DXA scan, OSA

(continued)

Table 2.1 (continued)

Disease name	Biochemical assessment	Clinical assessment
Alzheimer's disease and dementias	Alb, TTR, H&H, Gluc, Na^+, K^+, Fe^{2+}, Cu^{2+}, Zn, folate, vitamin B12, vitamin D, BUN, Creat, ALT, AST, CRP, Chol, choline acetyltransferase activity, dopamine, CSF biomarkers (Aβ42, total tau, phosphorylated tau), CSF pyruvate and lactate, tHcy	Bowel incontinence, history of Down syndrome, depression, history of herpes type 1 or HIV infection, loss of sense of smell
Schizophrenia	Alb, TTR, H&H, Gluc, Na^+, K^+, Ca^{2+}, Mg^{2+}, Fe^{2+}, ferritin, Chol, trig, insulin, CPK, folate, vitamin B12, vitamin D, Methylmalonic acid, MTHFR polymorphisms, VLDLR, mRNA levels	BP, sleep problems, anhedonia, flat affect, lack of motivation, global assessment of functioning scale, irritability
Parkinson's disease	Alb, TTR, H&H, Gluc, Na^+, K^+, Ca^{2+}, Mg^{2+}, Fe^{2+}, manganese, folate, vitamin B12, vitamin D, BUN, Creat, ALT, AST, dopamine, norepinephrine, tHcy, N balance, UA	Bradykinesia, depression or dementia, DXA scan, insomnia / rapid eye movement sleep disorder, postural instability or stooping, urinary frequency and urgency
Stroke	Alb, TTR, H&H, Gluc, Na^+, K^+, Ca^{2+}, Mg^{2+}, Fe^{2+}, ferritin, folate, Chol, HDL, LDL, trig, vitamin B12, CPK, LDH, CRP, vitamin D, PT, INR, tHcy, UA	BP, OSA, temperature, visual field scan
Multiple sclerosis	Alb, H&H, Gluc, Na^+, K^+, Fe^{2+}, Chol, trig, thyroid tests, vitamin B12, vitamin D, cerebrospinal fluid (CSF; WBC and γ-globulin), Osteopontin	BP, dizziness, Edema, temperature

(continued)

Table 2.1 (continued)

Disease name	Biochemical assessment	Clinical assessment
Guillain-Barré syndrome	Alb, TTR, Gluc, Fe^{2+}, CBC, vitamin D, CRP, lumbar puncture for CSF protein, pO_2, pCO_2, blood test for Zika or other viruses	BP, fatigue, weakness, fever, headache, joint or muscle pain, tingling in extremities

Abbreviations: Ca^{2+} (calcium), Mg^{2+} (magnesium), Na^+ (sodium), K^+ (potassium), Gluc (glucose), UA (uric acid), Chol (cholesterol), LDL (low-density lipoprotein), HDL (high-density lipoprotein), trig (triglycerides), Zn (zinc), tHcy (Total homocysteine), CBC (complete blood count), Alb (albumin), TTR (transthyretin), LFTs (liver function tests), RAST (Radioallergosorbent test), AlkP (alkaline phosphatase), H&H (Hemoglobin and Hematocrit), TFN (transferrin), CK (Creatine kinase), Cu^{2+} (copper), N balance (nitrogen balance), BUN (blood urea nitrogen), Creat (creatinine), ALT (alanine aminotransferase), AST (aspartate aminotransferase), CSF (cerebrospinal fluid), VLDLR (very low-density lipoprotein receptor), mRNA (messenger ribonucleic acid), PT (prothrombin time), INR (international normalized ratio), pO_2 (partial pressure of oxygen), pCO_2 (partial pressure of carbon dioxide), CRP (C-reactive protein), CPK (Creatine phosphokinase), MTHFR (methylenetetrahydrofolate reductase), IL-6 (Interleukin-6), TNF-α (tumor necrosis factor-alpha), LDH (lactate dehydrogenase), DXA (dual-energy X-ray absorptiometry), BP (blood pressure), OSA (obstructive sleep apnea)

2.3 Dietary Assessment

Dietary assessment is essential for evaluating nutritional status, especially in patients with disability disorders. Nutritional intake is estimated using a nutrition analysis program based on a food diary, 24-h recall, or food frequency questionnaire, with food diaries over three to seven days being the most reliable. Meal analysis provides insights into nutrient intake and recent eating patterns. Disability disorders can affect dietary intake through dysphagia, movement disorders, cognitive impairment, or depression, making accurate assessment crucial for planning effective nutritional interventions (Lee, 2022).

Acknowledgments The authors confirm that the content, analysis, and conclusions of this manuscript are their own work. AI-based tools were used solely to assist in improving the clarity and correctness of the English language.

References

Aborageh, M., Hähnel, T., Martins Conde, P., Klucken, J., & Fröhlich, H. (2025). Predicting dementia in people with Parkinson's disease. *npj Parkinson's Disease, 11*(1), 126.

Aging NIo. (2022). *Loss of smell linked to Alzheimer's cognitive impairment and biomarkers.* National Institute on Aging. https://www.nia.nih.gov/news/loss-smell-linked-alzheimers-cognitive-impairment-and-biomarkers?utm_source=chatgpt.com

Ahmed, G. K., Darwish, A. M., Khalifa, H., & Haridy, N. A. (2022). Relationship between attention deficit hyperactivity disorder and epilepsy: A literature review. *The Egyptian Journal of Neurology, Psychiatry and Neurosurgery., 58*(1), 52.

Ahuja, A., Martin, J., Langley, K., & Thapar, A. (2013). Intellectual disability in children with attention deficit hyperactivity disorder. *The Journal of Pediatrics, 163*(3), 890–5.e1.

Ballal, S. A., Greenwell, S., Liu, E., Buie, T., Silvester, J., Leier, M., et al. (2024). Comparing gastrointestinal endoscopy findings in children with autism, developmental delay, or typical development. *The Journal of Pediatrics, 264*, 113737.

Berardelli, A., Rothwell, J. C., Thompson, P. D., & Hallett, M. (2001). Pathophysiology of bradykinesia in Parkinson's disease. *Brain, 124*(Pt 11), 2131–2146.

Binda, D. D., Baker, M. B., Varghese, S., Wang, J., Badenes, R., Bilotta, F., et al. (2024). Targeted temperature management for patients with acute ischemic stroke: A literature review. *Journal of Clinical Medicine, 13*(2), 586.

Christogianni, A., Bibb, R., Davis, S. L., Jay, O., Barnett, M., Evangelou, N., et al. (2018). Temperature sensitivity in multiple sclerosis: An overview of its impact on sensory and cognitive symptoms. *Temperature, 5*(3), 208–223.

Cizza, G., Primma, S., Coyle, M., Gourgiotis, L., & Csako, G. (2010). Depression and osteoporosis: A research synthesis with meta-analysis. *Hormone and Metabolic Research, 42*(7), 467–482.

Cooper, M. S., Mackay, M. T., Dagia, C., Fahey, M. C., Howell, K. B., Reddihough, D., et al. (2023). Epilepsy syndromes in cerebral palsy: Varied, evolving and mostly self-limited. *Brain, 146*(2), 587–599.

Costi, S., Mecugni, D., Beccani, L., Alboresi, S., Bressi, B., Paltrinieri, S., et al. (2020). Construct validity of the activities scale for kids performance in children with cerebral palsy: Brief report. *Developmental Neurorehabilitation, 23*(7), 474–477.

De Georgia, M., Bowen, T., Duncan, K. R., & Chebl, A. B. (2023). Blood pressure management in ischemic stroke patients undergoing mechanical thrombectomy. *Neurological Research and Practice, 5*(1), 12.

de Gonzalo-Calvo, D., Barroeta, I., Nan, M. N., Rives, J., Garzón, D., Carmona-Iragui, M., et al. (2020). Evaluation of biochemical and hematological parameters in adults with Down syndrome. *Scientific Reports, 10*(1), 13755.

Deramore Denver, B., Froude, E., Rosenbaum, P., Wilkes-Gillan, S., & Imms, C. (2016). Measurement of visual ability in children with cerebral palsy: A systematic review. *Developmental Medicine and Child Neurology, 58*(10), 1016–1029.

Dorszewska, J., & Kozubski, W. (2016). Introductory chapter-genetic and biochemical factors. In *Challenges in Parkinson's disease* (p. 1).

Dyck, M. J., & Piek, J. P. (2014). Developmental delays in children with ADHD. *Journal of Attention Disorders, 18*(5), 466–478.

Farmakidis, C., Inan, S., Milstein, M., & Herskovitz, S. (2015). Headache and pain in Guillain-Barré syndrome. *Current Pain and Headache Reports, 19*(8), 40.

Fernando, T., & Goldman, R. D. (2019). Management of gastroesophageal reflux disease in pediatric patients with cerebral palsy. *Canadian Family Physician, 65*(11), 796–798.

Ferrarelli, F. (2021). Sleep abnormalities in schizophrenia: State of the art and next steps. *American Journal of Psychiatry, 178*(9), 903–913.

Fields, V. L., Soke, G. N., Reynolds, A., Tian, L. H., Wiggins, L., Maenner, M., et al. (2021). Pica, autism, and other disabilities. *Pediatrics, 147*(2), e20200462.

Fritz, M., Shenar, R., Cardenas-Morales, L., Jäger, M., Streb, J., Dudeck, M., et al. (2020). Aggressive and disruptive behavior among psychiatric patients with major depressive disorder, schizophrenia, or alcohol dependency and the effect of depression and self-esteem on aggression. *Frontiers in Psychiatry, 11*, 599828.

Fu, X., Wu, W., Wu, Y., Liu, X., Liang, W., Wu, R., et al. (2025). Adult ADHD and comorbid anxiety and depressive disorders: A review of etiology and treatment. *Frontiers in Psychiatry, 16*, 1597559.

Goffinski, A., Stanley, M. A., Shepherd, N., Duvall, N., Jenkinson, S. B., Davis, C., et al. (2015). Obstructive sleep apnea in young infants with Down syndrome evaluated in a Down syndrome specialty clinic. *American Journal of Medical Genetics. Part A, 167a*(2), 324–330.

Goodman, C., Rycroft Malone, J., Norton, C., Harari, D., Harwood, R., Roe, B., et al. (2015). Reducing and managing faecal incontinence in people with advanced dementia who are resident in care homes: Protocol for a realist synthesis. *BMJ Open, 5*(7), e007728.

Gur, R. E., Kohler, C. G., Ragland, J. D., Siegel, S. J., Lesko, K., Bilker, W. B., et al. (2006). Flat affect in schizophrenia: Relation to emotion processing and neurocognitive measures. *Schizophrenia Bulletin, 32*(2), 279–287.

Harale, M., Oommen, A., Faruqi, A., Mundada, M., Reddy, R. H., Pancholi, T., et al. (2024). Study of biochemical predictors of early neurological deterioration in ischemic stroke in a tertiary care hospital. *Cureus, 16*(8), e68183.

Horan, W. P., Kring, A. M., & Blanchard, J. J. (2006). Anhedonia in schizophrenia: A review of assessment strategies. *Schizophrenia Bulletin, 32*(2), 259–273.

Huang, Y.-Y., Gan, Y.-H., Yang, L., Cheng, W., & Yu, J.-T. (2024). Depression in Alzheimer's disease: Epidemiology, mechanisms, and treatment. *Biological Psychiatry, 95*(11), 992–1005.

Hurjui, I. A., Hurjui, R. M., Hurjui, L. L., Serban, I. L., Dobrin, I., Apostu, M., et al. (2025). Biomarkers and neuropsychological tools in attention-deficit/hyperactivity disorder: From subjectivity to precision diagnosis. *Medicina, 61*(7), 1211.

Hvolby, A. (2015). Associations of sleep disturbance with ADHD: Implications for treatment. *Atten Defic Hyperact Disord, 7*(1), 1–18.

Jehan, S., Farag, M., Zizi, F., Pandi-Perumal, S. R., Chung, A., Truong, A., et al. (2018). Obstructive sleep apnea and stroke. *Sleep Medicine and Disorders: International Journal, 2*(5), 120.

Kahle, S., Mukherjee, P., Dixon, J. F., Leibenluft, E., Hinshaw, S. P., & Schweitzer, J. B. (2021). Irritability predicts hyperactive/impulsive symptoms across adolescence for females. *Res Child Adolesc Psychopathol, 49*(2), 185–196.

Khandelwal, R., Manjunath, V. V., Mehta, L., & Mangajjera, S. B. (2023). Hematological and biochemical profiles in children with cerebral palsy: A cross-sectional study. *Journal of Pediatric Rehabilitation Medicine, 16*(1), 171–177.

Kim, C. S., Sung, Y. H., Kang, M. J., & Park, K. H. (2016). Rapid eye movement sleep behavior disorder in Parkinson's disease: A preliminary study. *Journal of Movement Disorders, 9*(2), 114–119.

Koga, M., Yuki, N., & Hirata, K. (2001). Antecedent symptoms in Guillain-Barré syndrome: An important indicator for clinical and serological subgroups. *Acta Neurologica Scandinavica, 103*(5), 278–287.

Köhler, O., Horsdal, H. T., Baandrup, L., Mors, O., & Gasse, C. (2016). Association between global assessment of functioning scores and indicators of functioning, severity, and prognosis in first-time schizophrenia. *Clinical Epidemiology, 8*, 323–332.

Kwok, M. K., & Schooling, C. M. (2021). Herpes simplex virus and Alzheimer's disease: A Mendelian randomization study. *Neurobiology of Aging, 99*(101), e11–e13.

Lan, Y.-L., & Chen, T.-L. (2012). Prevalence of high blood pressure and its relationship with body weight factors among inpatients with schizophrenia in Taiwan. *Asian Nursing Research, 6*(1), 13–18.

Latif, S. A. A., Hassan, H., Ibrahim, O., Fotouh, A. E. A. E., Mohamed, M. O., & Tantawy, A. M. E. (2024). Comorbidity of depression and anxiety with obstructive sleep apnea in a sample of Egyptian patients. *Middle East Current Psychiatry, 31*(1), 29.

Lee, B. J. (2021). Association of depressive disorder with biochemical and anthropometric indices in adult men and women. *Scientific Reports, 11*(1), 13596.

Lee, H. (2022). The importance of nutrition in neurological disorders and nutrition assessment methods. *Brain Neurorehabil, 15*(1), e1.

Li, X., Mao, Y., Zhu, S., Ma, J., Gao, S., Jin, X., et al. (2023). Relationship between depressive disorders and biochemical indicators in adult men and women. *BMC Psychiatry, 23*(1), 49.

Luft, V. C., Beghetto, M. G., Castro, S. M., & de Mello, E. D. (2008). Validation of a new method developed to measure the height of adult patients in bed. *Nutrition in Clinical Practice, 23*(4), 424–428.

Malak, R., Kostiukow, A., Krawczyk-Wasielewska, A., Mojs, E., & Samborski, W. (2015). Delays in motor development in children with Down syndrome. *Medical Science Monitor, 21*, 1904–1910.

Mark, M., & Duff, E. (2023). Primary care management of hypertension in patients with multiple sclerosis. *The Journal for Nurse Practitioners, 19*(7), 104652.

Marsh, L. (2013). Depression and Parkinson's disease: Current knowledge. *Current Neurology and Neuroscience Reports, 13*(12), 409.

Maure-Blesa, L., Carmona-Iragui, M., Lott, I., Head, E., Wisniewski, T., Rafii, M. S., et al. (2025). The history of Down syndrome-associated Alzheimer's disease; past, present, and future. *Alzheimer's & Dementia, 21*(6), e70158.

Meena, A., Khadilkar, S., & Murthy, J. (2011). Treatment guidelines for Guillain–Barré syndrome. *Annals of Indian Academy of Neurology, 14*(Suppl1), S73–S81.

MHDSA. (2024). *Protruding tongue Down syndrome*. Retrieved August 9, 2024, from https://www.mhdsa.org/protruding-tongue-down-syndrome/

Nayak, A. R., Kashyap, R. S., Kabra, D., Deoras, P., Purohit, H. J., Taori, G. M., et al. (2011). Evaluation of routinely performed hematological and biochemical parameters for the prognosis of acute ischemic stroke patients. *Neurological Sciences, 32*(5), 855–860.

Niedziela, N., Pierzchała, K., Zalejska-Fiolka, J., Niedziela, J. T., Romuk, E., Torbus-Paluszczak, M., et al. (2018). Assessment of biochemical and densitometric markers of calcium-phosphate metabolism in the groups of patients with multiple sclerosis selected due to the serum level of vitamin D3. *BioMed Research International, 2018*(1), 9329123.

Nikouei Moghaddam, M. R., Movahedi, M., Bananej, M., Najafi, S., Moghadam, N. B., Saadat, P., et al. (2021). Assessment of biochemical determinants in multiple sclerosis patients following the oral administration of β-D-Mannuronic acid (M2000). *Current Drug Discovery Technologies, 18*(5), e17092020186049.

Nurković, J. S., Petković, P., Tiosavljević, D., & Vojinović, R. (2020). Measurement of bone mineral density in children with cerebral palsy from an ethical issue to a diagnostic necessity. *BioMed Research International, 2020*, 7282946.

Palakurthi, B., & Burugupally, S. P. (2019). Postural instability in Parkinson's disease: A review. *Brain Sciences, 9*(9), 239.

Paneyala, S., Naseer, A., Iyer, M., & Gopi, A. (2024). Assessment of serum inflammatory markers and their correlation with clinical severity and electrophysiological subtypes of Guillain Barre syndrome, and investigating their use as prognostic markers of Guillain Barre syndrome. *Annals of Indian Academy of Neurology, 27*(1), 101–103.

Parker, A. W., & James, B. (1985). Age changes in the flexibility of down's syndrome children. *Journal of Mental Deficiency Research, 29*(Pt 3), 207–218.

Polat, I. E., Kuzay, D., & Konar, N. M. (2021). Analysing biochemical parameters and developing risk prediction models in patients with schizophrenia and bipolar disorder. *Electronic Journal of Medical and Educational Technologies, 14*(3), em2112.

Rabbito, A., Dulewicz, M., Kulczyńska-Przybik, A., & Mroczko, B. (2020). Biochemical markers in Alzheimer's disease. *International Journal of Molecular Sciences, 21*(6), 1989.

Ranjani, P., Khanna, M., Gupta, A., Nagappa, M., Taly, A. B., & Haldar, P. (2014). Prevalence of fatigue in Guillain-Barre syndrome in neurological rehabilitation setting. *Annals of Indian Academy of Neurology, 17*(3), 331–335.

Roberts, J. R., Dawley, E. H., & Reigart, J. R. (2019). Children's low-level pesticide exposure and associations with autism and ADHD: A review. *Pediatric Research, 85*(2), 234–241.

S E-S. (2022). *Nutrition & diagnosis-related care* (9th ed.). Academy of Nutrition and Dietetics.

Salman, A., Islam, S., Saleh, M. A., Bhinder, K. K., Malik, Z., Tahir, I., et al. (2021). Retracted: Nutritional and biochemical parameters among multiple sclerosis patients: A case-control study. *Cureus, 13*(5), r31.

Salvatore Orefice, N., Ferraro, O., Barbato, F., Carotenuto, A., Lanzillo, R., Brescia Morra, V., et al. (2012). Biochemical parameters alterations in multiple sclerosis: A longitudinal study and review of the literature. *Pharmacology & Pharmacy, 3*(02), 248–253.

Sand, K. M., Thomassen, L., Næss, H., Rødahl, E., & Hoff, J. M. (2012). Diagnosis and rehabilitation of visual field defects in stroke patients: A retrospective audit. *Cerebrovascular Diseases Extra, 2*(1), 17–23.

Sarathy, K., Doshi, C., & Aroojis, A. (2019). Clinical examination of children with cerebral palsy. *Indian Journal of Orthopaedics, 53*(1), 35–44.

Senarathne, U. D., Indika, N. R., Jezela-Stanek, A., Ciara, E., Frye, R. E., Chen, C., et al. (2023). Biochemical, genetic and clinical diagnostic approaches to autism-associated inherited metabolic disorders. *Genes (Basel), 14*(4), 803.

Society NMS. (2025). *Vertigo & dizziness*. https://www.nationalmssociety.org/understanding-ms/what-is-ms/ms-symptoms/vertigo-dizziness

Solaro, C., Messmer Uccelli, M., Brichetto, G., Augello, G., Taddei, G., Boccardo, F., et al. (2006). Prevalence of oedema of the lower limbs in multiple sclerosis patients: A vascular and lymphoscintigraphic study. *Multiple Sclerosis, 12*(5), 659–661.

Solomon, B. D., Balachandar, D., Perry, K., Carrillo-Carrasco, N., Markello, T. C., & Rais-Bahrami, K. (2008). Trisomy 21 in one of extremely low birth weight twins. *Journal of Neonatal-Perinatal Medicine, 1*(3), 193–196.

Soryal, I., Sinclair, E., Hornby, J., & Pentland, B. (1992). Impaired joint mobility in Guillain-Barré syndrome: A primary or a secondary phenomenon? *Journal of Neurology, Neurosurgery, and Psychiatry, 55*(11), 1014–1017.

Stroke NIoNDa. (2025). *Guillain-Barré syndrome*. https://www.ninds.nih.gov/health-information/disorders/guillain-barre-syndrome

Team FC. (2025). *Biochemical and clinical markers of nutritional status*. Fiveable. https://fiveable.me/advanced-nutrition/unit-10/biochemical-clinical-markers-nutritional-status/study-guide/ELmbL02UC3SpHRSb?utm_source=chatgpt.com

Torsney, K. M., Noyce, A. J., Doherty, K. M., Bestwick, J. P., Dobson, R., & Lees, A. J. (2014). Bone health in Parkinson's disease: A systematic review and meta-analysis. *Journal of Neurology, Neurosurgery & Psychiatry, 85*(10), 1159–1166.

Waltz, J. A., & Gold, J. M. (2015). Motivational deficits in schizophrenia and the representation of expected value. *Behavioral Neuroscience of Motivation, 27*, 375–410.

Wang, Z., Xia, H., Shi, J., Fan, P., Cao, Q., Ding, Y., et al. (2024). Investigating the genetic association of 40 biochemical indicators with Parkinson's disease. *Journal of Molecular Neuroscience, 74*(4), 92.

Yahya, A. F., Haddad, N. I., & Saud, A. M. (2023). Assessment of serum neuron specific enolase (NSE) and other biochemical parameters in Iraqi patients with ischemic stroke. *The Egyptian Journal of Hospital Medicine, 91*(1), 5162–5168.

Yeo, L., Singh, R., Gundeti, M., Barua, J. M., & Masood, J. (2012). Urinary tract dysfunction in Parkinson's disease: A review. *International Urology and Nephrology, 44*(2), 415–424.

Chapter 3
Down Syndrome

Abstract

- Down syndrome (DS), caused by trisomy 21, is the most common chromosomal disorder leading to intellectual disability and is characterized by hypotonia, dysmorphic features, short stature, and congenital heart disease.
- The incidence of DS ranges from 1 in 319 to 1 in 1000 live births and increases with maternal age, while clinical manifestations vary widely, and early healthcare interventions improve developmental outcomes.
- DS primarily results from nondisjunction during gamete formation, with risk factors including advanced maternal age, parental chromosomal translocations, and a previously affected child, making genetic counseling important for high-risk families.
- Nutritional management is essential for promoting growth, supporting development, and preventing obesity, diabetes, and cardiovascular disease, as individuals with DS often experience slower metabolism, feeding difficulties, gastrointestinal disorders, and food selectivity.
- Nutrition-related challenges such as overweight, obesity, type 1 and 2 diabetes, celiac disease, constipation, gastroesophageal reflux, and heart defects require individualized dietary adaptation, monitoring, and multidisciplinary support.
- Medical nutrition therapy emphasizes nutrient-dense diets with adequate energy, protein, complex carbohydrates, healthy fats, fiber, and micronutrients including vitamins A, C, D, E, B-complex, zinc, and selenium.
- Growth monitoring should use DS-specific charts, assess thyroid function, iron, vitamin D, and glucose, and follow pediatric dietary guidelines adapted to DS-specific comorbidities.
- Awareness of food–drug interactions and coordinated multidisciplinary care further optimize health, development, and quality of life in individuals with DS.

Keywords Down syndrome (DS) · Chromosomal disorders · Intellectual disability · Nutrition · Feeding difficulties · Obesity · Gastrointestinal disorders · Micronutrients · Growth monitoring · Food–drug interactions

M. H. Rouhani et al., *The Healing Plate*, SpringerBriefs in Modern Perspectives on Disability Research, https://doi.org/10.1007/978-981-95-8150-4_3

3.1 Definition and Epidemiology

Down syndrome (DS) is the most common chromosomal disability disorder among liveborn infants, resulting from the presence of an extra chromosome 21 (trisomy 21). It represents the leading chromosomal cause of intellectual disability and is associated with a wide spectrum of physical characteristics and medical complications, including distinctive dysmorphic features, hypotonia, joint laxity, short stature, and congenital heart disease. Clinical presentation is highly variable, as not all features occur in every affected individual (Akhtar & Bokhari, 2020; Roizen & Patterson, 2003; Weijerman & De Winter, 2010).

The incidence of DS shows considerable variation across populations, ranging from approximately 1 in 319 to 1 in 1000 live births, and increases significantly with advancing maternal age. Although the conception rate of fetuses with trisomy 21 is relatively high, an estimated 50–75% are lost before term. In comparison, other autosomal trisomies occur more frequently at conception, but their survival beyond birth is markedly lower. The relatively higher postnatal survival of individuals with trisomy 21 has been attributed to the limited number of genes located on chromosome 21 (Hsa21), which is the smallest and least gene-dense of the autosomes (Asim et al., 2015; Bittles & Glasson, 2004; Roper & Reeves, 2006).

The clinical manifestations of DS are diverse and vary among individuals, with different problems potentially arising at different stages of life. Common physical features include hypotonia, short neck with excess skin folds, flattened facial profile, small head, ears, and mouth, upward slanting eyes often with epicanthal folds, Brushfield spots, broad short hands with a single palmar crease, and a wide gap between the first and second toes. Physical development is typically delayed, and children may achieve motor milestones such as sitting, standing, or walking later than peers, although most eventually attain them (Antonarakis et al., 2020; Bull & Genetics Co, 2011; Estigarribia, 2025; Ulrich et al., 2011).

3.2 Etiology

DS results from a random error in cell division, most commonly nondisjunction, where both copies of chromosome 21 fail to separate and migrate into the same cell. This leads to an extra copy of chromosome 21 in each cell. The error usually occurs during the formation of the egg or sperm, and current evidence does not implicate any parental behavior or environmental factor as a cause.

Although the exact cause of DS is not fully understood, several risk factors have been identified. The most significant is maternal age, as the likelihood of abnormal chromosomal division increases with age, particularly after 35 years. Parental genetic factors also play a role; parents who carry a chromosomal translocation involving chromosome 21 or who have previously had a child with DS are at higher risk of recurrence. Genetic counseling is recommended for such families (Allen et al., 2009; Coppedè, 2016; Ghosh et al., 2009; Morris et al., 2005; Sherman et al., 2007).

3.3 Nutritional Management

Nutrition plays a crucial role in promoting health, growth, and development in individuals with DS. A well-balanced and varied diet provides the necessary energy and nutrients for daily activities, helps maintain a healthy weight, and reduces the risk of long-term health problems such as type 2 diabetes, cardiovascular disease, and obesity (Irish Nutrition & Dietetic Institute (INDI), 2023).

3.3.1 Nutrition-Related Challenges

Children and adults with DS are at increased risk for certain nutrition-related concerns. A slower metabolism makes them more prone to weight gain as well as increasing their susceptibility to obesity-related complications. Gastrointestinal issues, such as celiac disease, can affect nutrient absorption, and oral–motor or sensory difficulties may interfere with chewing, swallowing, and safe feeding. Early nutritional assessment and consultation with feeding specialists are important to ensure adequate nutrient intake, support optimal growth, and improve overall quality of life (Nordstrøm et al., 2020; Ravel et al., 2020; Żur et al., 2025).

Overweight and Obesity

Overweight and obesity are prevalent health concerns among individuals with DS, requiring a comprehensive and individualized management approach that integrates nutritional and physical activity strategies. Contributing factors include hypothyroidism, hormonal imbalances, low muscle tone (leading to higher fat mass and lower muscle mass), reduced physical activity, poor dietary habits, sleep disturbances, certain medications, and behavioral factors such as emotional eating. These issues increase the risk of secondary complications, including type 2 diabetes, cardiovascular disease, sleep apnea, gastroesophageal reflux, arthritis, and aspiration pneumonia. A thorough clinical and dietary assessment is essential to identify underlying causes and behavioral triggers, followed by collaboration with healthcare providers to monitor weight and implement evidence-based interventions (National Down Syndrome Society, n.d.; National Center on Health PAaDN, n.d.;

Illinois Department of Central Management Services / Be Well Illinois, n.d.). Practical recommendations for addressing these challenges are summarized in Box 3.1.

Box 3.1 Key Recommendations for Weight Management

- Provide a balanced diet with controlled portion sizes.
- Emphasize fruits, vegetables, whole grains, lean protein, and low-fat dairy.
- Limit processed foods and sugar-sweetened beverages.
- Encourage small, frequent meals instead of irregular grazing.
- Promote adequate hydration with water as the main beverage.
- Aim for 15–30 min of moderate physical activity daily, tailored to ability.
- Screen regularly for hypothyroidism and review medications that may contribute to weight gain.
- Identify emotional and behavioral triggers for overeating and address them through structured routines.
- Involve caregivers and family in meal planning, grocery shopping, and food preparation.
- Use tracking tools or visual aids to monitor eating habits and progress.
- Monitor weight trends and adjust nutritional and activity plans as needed.

Diabetes

Individuals with DS have a higher prevalence of type 1 diabetes compared to the general population and may also face an elevated risk of developing type 2 diabetes due to the increased rates of obesity and other metabolic risk factors. Type 1 diabetes often presents in childhood, making early recognition essential. Common symptoms include increased thirst, frequent urination, unexplained weight loss, and fatigue.

Nutrition plays a central role in the management of both type 1 and type 2 diabetes, alongside medication and regular monitoring of blood glucose levels. Comprehensive diabetes education for caregivers and individuals with DS is recommended to support effective management strategies, including balanced dietary planning, portion control, and appropriate carbohydrate distribution. Consulting a registered dietitian or certified diabetes educator is strongly advised to ensure individualized care (National Down Syndrome Society, n.d.; National Center on Health PAaDN, n.d.; Whooten et al., 2018).

Celiac Disease

Individuals with DS have a significantly higher prevalence of celiac disease, with incidence estimates ranging from 7% to 16%, compared to the general population. Celiac disease is an autoimmune disorder triggered by the ingestion of gluten, a protein found in wheat, barley, and rye. In affected individuals, gluten consumption leads to an immune-mediated injury of the small intestinal mucosa, resulting in malabsorption and nutritional deficiencies.

Clinical manifestations can vary and may include poor weight gain, chronic diarrhea, vomiting, constipation, behavioral changes, and signs of nutrient deficiency. Screening is often initiated with a simple serological blood test, while a definitive diagnosis requires confirmatory evaluation by a gastroenterology specialist.

The cornerstone of treatment is lifelong adherence to a strict gluten-free diet, completely eliminating wheat, barley, and rye. Dietary management should emphasize naturally gluten-free whole foods such as fruits, vegetables, legumes, quinoa, and brown rice to ensure adequate fiber and micronutrient intake while maintaining nutritional adequacy (National Down Syndrome Society, n.d.; National Center on Health PAaDN, n.d.; Cogulu et al., 2003). A cardioprotective gluten-free diet should be prescribed for these patients (Fig. 3.1).

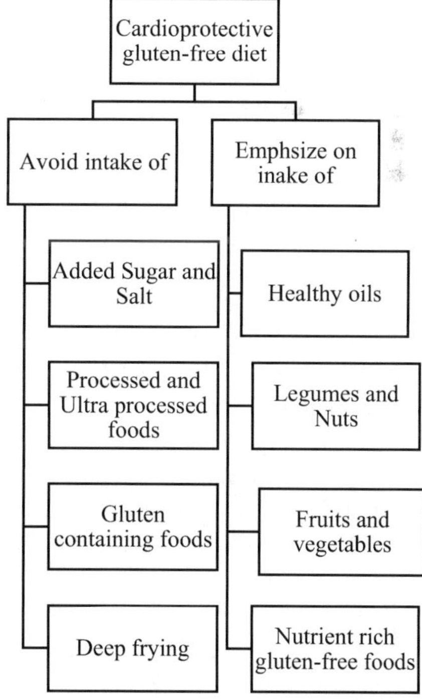

Fig. 3.1 A cardioprotective gluten-free diet

Constipation

Constipation is a frequent concern in individuals with DS, largely due to low muscle tone, sedentary lifestyle, and dietary factors. Management should emphasize hydration, adequate fiber intake, proper toilet habits, and physical activity (National Center on Health PAaDN, n.d.; Rogers et al., n.d.). Key evidence-based strategies for prevention and treatment are summarized in Box 3.2.

Box 3.2 Key Recommendations for Constipation Prevention and Management

- **Hydration:** Encourage six to eight glasses of water daily.
- **Fiber Intake:** Include fruits and vegetables (with skin), dried fruits such as raisins, prunes, and figs, and whole-grain cereals.
- **Meal Pattern:** Offer small, frequent meals to support bowel regularity.
- **Toilet Training:** Promote proper posture and routine toileting habits.
- **Physical Stimulation:** Use abdominal massage, leg cycling, and blowing games.
- **Probiotics:** Add to diet as supportive therapy.
- **Medical Support:** Consult a dietitian or physician for persistent constipation; consider fiber supplements when necessary.

Gastroesophageal Reflux Disease

Gastroesophageal Reflux Disease (GERD) occurs when stomach contents flow back into the esophagus, causing symptoms such as heartburn, regurgitation, sore throat, hoarseness, chest pain, cough, and occasionally difficulty swallowing. GERD is more common in individuals with DS and may go undiagnosed, particularly in those with communication difficulties. Contributing factors can include obesity, overeating, sleep apnea, gallstones, or sometimes no identifiable cause. Chronic untreated GERD can affect nutrient intake and oral health, including tooth enamel erosion.

Dietary and lifestyle strategies are essential for reducing GERD symptoms and improving quality of life. The following recommendations are suggested:

- Eat small, frequent meals rather than large ones.
- Practice portion control at meals and snacks.
- Avoid lying down for at least 2–3 h after eating.
- Drink fluids between meals instead of during meals.
- Wait at least 1 h after eating before exercising.
- Limit or avoid trigger foods such as acidic foods (tomato, citrus), fried or fatty foods, processed meats, caffeine, chocolate, spicy foods, and carbonated beverages.

- Maintain a healthy weight to reduce abdominal pressure.
- Elevate the head and upper body during sleep if reflux occurs at night.
- Wear loose-fitting clothing to avoid pressure on the abdomen.
- Seek medical evaluation if symptoms persist, as pharmacological management may be necessary (National Center on Health PAaDN, n.d.; Down's Syndrome Medical Interest Group (DSMIG)., 2020).

Heart Defects

Cardiovascular disease is one of the leading causes of morbidity and mortality in people with DS. Congenital heart disease (CHD) is the most common cardiovascular abnormality, affecting up to 50% of individuals with DS. Other contributing factors to cardiovascular complications include pulmonary hypertension, endocrine and metabolic disorders, and increased risk for atherosclerotic disease.

Nutritional management plays a critical role in both early care and long-term prevention of cardiovascular complications. In newborns with severe heart defects, nutrition support or temporary tube feeding may be required before and after surgery to ensure adequate growth and recovery. As children grow, and into adulthood, following a heart-healthy dietary pattern is essential. Key recommendations include:

- Prioritize a diet rich in fruits, vegetables, whole grains, and dietary fiber.
- Include lean protein sources such as poultry, fish, legumes, and low-fat dairy.
- Ensure adequate hydration, preferably with water.
- Limit processed and fried foods, foods high in saturated or trans fats, sugar-sweetened beverages, sweets, and excessive salt intake.
- Encourage maintaining a healthy weight through balanced nutrition and physical activity as advised by the healthcare team (National Center on Health PAaDN, n.d.; Dimopoulos et al., 2023).
- **Feeding Difficulties and Food Selectivity.**

Feeding difficulties are highly prevalent in children with DS, especially during infancy. These challenges are often multifactorial, related to hypotonia, oral–motor incoordination, altered sensory perception, narrow palate, and associated medical conditions such as gastroesophageal reflux, congenital heart disease, prematurity, and respiratory disorders. In some cases, cow's milk protein intolerance may also contribute. More than half of children with DS experience silent aspiration, which can go undetected without careful assessment.

Most feeding challenges can be addressed conservatively using a multidisciplinary approach involving speech and language therapists, dietitians, occupational therapists, and pediatricians. Management strategies include:

- Routine assessment of feeding and swallowing at each clinic visit during infancy, with further evaluation if aspiration is suspected.

- Adjusting food textures to ensure safe swallowing, gradually progressing toward a regular texture diet as skills improve.
- Encouraging and supporting mothers who wish to breastfeed.
- Temporary nasogastric or nasojejunal feeding may be necessary during infancy, especially when medical complications are present; long-term gastrostomy is rarely required.
- Introducing new foods slowly and without pressure, recognizing that more than 20 exposures may be needed before acceptance.
- Working with a feeding team to develop individualized strategies that address sensory preferences and oral–motor challenges.
- Engaging caregivers in meal preparation and feeding routines to create a positive and supportive environment (National Down Syndrome Society, n.d.; National Center on Health PAaDN, n.d.; Down Syndrome Medical Interest Group (DSMIG), 2022).

3.3.2 Medical Nutrition Therapy

Medical nutrition therapy plays a key role in promoting health, supporting growth, and preventing complications in individuals with DS. Although there are no specific nutrient requirements unique to this population, studies have shown several dietary irregularities, including inadequate intake of fruits, vegetables, wholegrain cereals, and dairy products, as well as excessive consumption of meat products and sweets. These findings underscore the need to correct eating habits and follow balanced dietary recommendations similar to those for the general population, while also addressing health conditions more common in individuals with DS.

Clinical nutrition care should be individualized, multidisciplinary, and proactive. Regular assessments of growth patterns, feeding abilities, and biochemical markers are crucial to ensure optimal nutritional status. Dietitians should play a central role in both early intervention and ongoing management throughout life.

Energy and Macronutrients Requirements

Individuals with DS generally have a lower basal metabolic rate compared to the general population, meaning they burn approximately 10–15% fewer calories at rest. This reduction in energy expenditure, combined with factors such as reduced lean body mass, muscle hypotonia, and lower physical activity levels, increases the risk of excessive weight gain even when energy intake is only moderately elevated. To provide adequate energy according to age, children aged 5–11 years require 14.3 kcal per centimeter of height for girls and 16.1 kcal per centimeter of height for boys.

Because energy needs are lower, total caloric intake should be carefully monitored and typically remain slightly below the recommended daily allowance for individuals of the same age and height without DS. At the same time, nutritional quality must be preserved; nutrient density of foods becomes critical to ensure that vitamin, mineral, and macronutrient needs are still met despite a reduced total calorie intake. Using tools such as the food pyramid or MyPlate guidelines can help optimize food selection and maintain this delicate balance between adequate nutrient intake and weight management. This point should be taken into account that for individuals with underweight, energy intake should be individualized and increased cautiously, with attention to any underlying medical conditions contributing to weight loss or poor growth (Bertapelli et al., 2016; Down Syndrome Australia, 2015; Luke et al., 1996).

Protein plays an important role in growth, tissue repair, and the proper functioning of the immune system, making it a key macronutrient for children and adults with DS. Protein requirements for individuals with DS are generally consistent with those recommended for the general population and should come from varied sources of both plant and animal origin.

In cases of malnutrition or excess body weight, protein intake may need to be increased to support adequate growth, preserve lean body mass, and promote healthy weight management. Each meal should ideally include a source of high-quality protein, with an emphasis on diversified sources from both animal and plant origins. Animal proteins provide essential amino acids and important micronutrients, including vitamin B12, which is crucial for preventing macrocytic anemia (Białek-Dratwa et al., 2022; Gruszka & Włodarek, 2024; Nordstrøm et al., 2020).

The primary sources of carbohydrates in the diet of individuals with DS should be complex carbohydrates, including whole grain cereals, and legumes. These foods help maintain a healthy body weight and support the prevention of metabolic disorders.

Simple sugars should be limited according to general population guidelines, with particular attention in individuals with excess weight, prediabetes, or diabetes, where total carbohydrate intake may need further restriction.

Dietary fiber is an essential part of the diet. Recommendations include approximately 5–6 g of fiber per year of age per day for children over 3 years, and 25–30 g per day for adults. Fiber intake may need to be adjusted in the presence of gastrointestinal diseases such as intestinal inflammation, liver, stomach, or pancreatic disorders (Gruszka & Włodarek, 2024; Żur et al., 2025).

Fat intake in individuals with DS should be carefully managed. In some cases, such as those with liver or pancreatic conditions, total fat consumption may need to be reduced compared to the dietary recommendations. In addition, due to the elevated risk of cardiovascular disease and the presence of oxidative stress, dietary strategies should focus on limiting saturated fatty acids while ensuring adequate intake of monounsaturated and polyunsaturated fats, with particular emphasis on omega-3 fatty acids.

Although direct evidence is limited, children with DS are believed to exhibit early lipid metabolism abnormalities, including elevated LDL cholesterol and triglyceride levels, sometimes even in preschool age. Long-chain omega-3 fatty acids, especially eicosapentaenoic acid (EPA) and docosahexaenoic acid (DHA), are essential components of a diet that supports neurological development and immune function. DHA, a major structural element of the brain and retina, may contribute to cognitive development, visual function, and the regulation of inflammatory processes, which can be exacerbated in DS. Both EPA and DHA also provide anti-inflammatory and cardioprotective effects, addressing the heightened cardiovascular risk and immune dysregulation observed in this population.

Although well-controlled interventional studies in children with DS are still limited, current evidence suggests that including dietary sources of long-chain omega-3 fatty acids may offer significant health benefits, particularly during periods of rapid neurodevelopment or in the presence of inflammatory or autoimmune conditions (Gruszka & Włodarek, 2024; Shahidi & Ambigaipalan, 2018; Żur et al., 2025).

Micronutrients Requirements

Individuals with DS experience increased oxidative stress due to overexpression of several genes on chromosome 21, which is considered an important factor contributing to cognitive impairment and neurodegenerative changes characteristic of the syndrome. For this reason, their diet should be rich in antioxidants, including vitamins A, C, and E as well as minerals such as selenium and zinc, to help delay aging processes and the onset of chronic diseases.

Adequate intake of B vitamins, particularly folate, vitamin B6, and vitamin B12, is important due to the possible presence of folate metabolism polymorphisms, hyper-homocysteinemia, and impaired DNA methylation that may contribute to neurological complications, atherosclerosis, congenital heart defects, and hypothyroidism. Vitamin D and calcium should also be prioritized, with supplementation considered when deficiencies are present or when dairy intake is limited (Albu et al., 2022; Lyon et al., 2020; Rueda Revilla & Martínez-Cué, 2020; Shirode et al., 2023; Vraneković et al., 2020).

Zinc is the most frequently studied trace element in DS, and some studies suggest a risk of deficiency in this population. When deficiencies are suspected or confirmed, supplementation may be warranted, but any vitamin or mineral supplement should be introduced under the guidance of a qualified health professional.

Routine monitoring of thyroid function is recommended for infants and children with DS at birth and annually thereafter. Studies on zinc, copper, and selenium status generally indicate that deficiencies are not common when food access and appetite are adequate, highlighting the importance of regular growth monitoring and nutritional assessment (Barišić et al., 2023; Lima et al., 2010; Saghazadeh et al., 2017).

Dietary Guidelines and Therapeutic Approaches

Although research on the health and nutritional needs of children with DS has expanded considerably, no formal, standardized dietary guideline specific to DS has yet been established. In practice, clinicians and dietitians usually apply general pediatric dietary recommendations, tailoring them to the individual's health status and comorbid conditions such as congenital heart disease, gastrointestinal problems, or feeding difficulties. Several professional documents, however, serve as key reference frameworks for guiding nutritional care.

Guidance from the American Academy of Pediatrics (AAP).

The AAP clinical report "Health Supervision for Children and Adolescents with Down Syndrome" remains the most comprehensive source of recommendations for the overall care of children with DS. Although it does not dedicate a separate section exclusively to nutrition, it highlights several nutrition-related priorities:

- Monitoring growth using DS–specific growth charts (https://www.cdc.gov/birth-defects/hcp/down-syndrome-growth-charts/index.html).
- Performing regular laboratory evaluations, including iron, ferritin, vitamin D, thyroid function (TSH), and glucose levels.
- Encouraging healthy lifestyle habits, with emphasis on regular physical activity.
- Implementing early dietary interventions to manage or prevent malnutrition, overweight, and obesity.
- Referring to a clinical dietitian in cases of feeding disorders, gastrointestinal conditions, abnormal weight gain, or when an elimination diet is necessary.

This report strongly promotes a team-based, multidisciplinary approach to optimize care (Bull et al., 2022).

Recommendations from ESPGHAN and EFAD

Although ESPGHAN (European Society for Paediatric Gastroenterology, Hepatology and Nutrition) and EFAD (European Federation of Associations of Dietitians) have not issued DS-specific guidelines, their 2017 consensus on nutrition for children with neurological and developmental disorders provides principles that can be directly applied to the DS population:

- Adjusting total caloric intake according to the child's physical activity level and developmental stage, with an emphasis on preventing excess weight gain.
- Enhancing nutrient density when overall calorie intake is reduced.
- Monitoring growth routinely and adapting food texture and consistency to oral–motor capacity.
- Performing a comprehensive nutritional assessment (growth, biochemical markers, and feeding history) before planning interventions.
- Using a multidisciplinary team approach, involving physicians, dietitians, feeding specialists, physiotherapists, and psychologists (Romano et al., 2017).

Table 3.1 Commonly prescribed medications for cerebral palsy and their food–drug interactions

Drug	Trade Name	Food–Drug Interactions
Anticonvulsants		
Carbamazepine	Tegretol	**Side effects:** Weight gain and causes nutrient depletions (folic acid, biotin, and vitamin D) **Avoid:** St John's wort, grapefruit juice, pomegranate juice, and alcohol
Valproic acid	Depakote, Depakene	**Side effects:** Increased appetite, causes nutrient depletions (zinc—selenium—folic acid—vitamin B3 deficiencies) **Avoid:** Alcohol
Phenytoin	Dilantin	**Side effects:** Causes nutrient depletions (hypocalcemia, folic acid—vitamin B1—vitamin B12—vitamin K deficiencies), increases use of vitamin D in the body **Avoid:** Alcohol
Antidysrhythmic		
Digoxin	Lanoxin	**Side effects:** Causes nutrient depletions (hypocalcemia, hypomagnesemia, hypophosphatemia, hypokalemia, vitamin B1 deficiency) **Avoid:** Fiber-rich meals, St John's wort, Seville orange juice, panax ginseng
Diuretics		
Furosemide	Lasix	**Side effects:** Causes nutrient depletions (hypocalcemia, hypokalemia, hypomagnesemia **Avoid:** Alcohol
Hydrochlorothiazide	Esidrix	**Side effects:** Causes nutrient depletions (hypomagnesemia, hypokalemia, zinc deficiency) **Avoid:** High-carbohydrate meals, sodium in foods, alcohol
Metolazone	Zaroxolyn	**Side effects:** – **Avoid:** Alcohol
Others		
Rivastigmine	Exelon	**Side effects:** Anorexia **Avoid:** Alcohol
Galantamine	Razadyne	**Side effects:** Anorexia **Avoid:** Alcohol
Memantine	Namenda	**Side effects:** Anorexia **Avoid:** Alcohol
Donepezil	Aricept	**Side effects:** Anorexia **Avoid:** Alcohol
Levothyroxine	Synthroid	**Side effects:** – **Avoid:** Grapefruit juice, using multivitamin with minerals
Metformin	Glucophage	**Side effects:** Causes nutrient depletions (vitamin B12 deficiency) **Avoid:** Alcohol
L-methylfolate	Deplin	**Side effects:** – **Avoid:** Alcohol

3.4 Food and Drug Interaction

Drug therapy is not currently considered part of the standard treatment for DS, as there is no medication that can correct trisomy 21 itself. However, many individuals with DS are prescribed medications or supplements to manage associated health conditions. For example, thyroid hormone replacement is commonly recommended for hypothyroidism, which frequently occurs in this population (Angelakou, n.d.; Hefti & Blanco, 2017; Palumbo & McDougle, 2018). The most common medication that are used in DS along with their food–drug interaction illustrated in Table 3.1.

Acknowledgments The authors confirm that the content, analysis, and conclusions of this manuscript are their own work. AI-based tools were used solely to assist in improving the clarity and correctness of the English language.

References

Akhtar, F., & Bokhari, S. R. A. (2020). *Down syndrome (trisomy 21)*. StatPearls. https://www.ncbi.nlm.nih.gov/books/NBK526016/

Albu, C.-C., Russu, E., Albu, D., & Albu, Ş.-D. (2022). Folic acid and its implications in genetic pathology. *World Journal of Advanced Research and Reviews, 16*, 742–748.

Allen, E. G., Freeman, S. B., Druschel, C., Hobbs, C. A., O'Leary, L. A., Romitti, P. A., et al. (2009). Maternal age and risk for trisomy 21 assessed by the origin of chromosome nondisjunction: A report from the Atlanta and National Down Syndrome Projects. *Human Genetics, 125*(1), 41–52.

Angelakou, I. A. (n.d.). *Food-drug interactions and their impact on the pharmacotherapy*.

Antonarakis, S. E., Skotko, B. G., Rafii, M. S., Strydom, A., Pape, S. E., Bianchi, D. W., et al. (2020). Down syndrome. *Nature Reviews Disease Primers, 6*(1), 9.

Asim, A., Kumar, A., Muthuswamy, S., Jain, S., & Agarwal, S. (2015). Down syndrome: An insight of the disease. *Journal of Biomedical Science, 22*(1), 41.

Barišić, A., Ravančić, M., Majstorivić, D., & Vraneković, J. (2023). Micronutrient status in children and adolescents with Down syndrome: Systematic review and meta-analysis. *Journal of Intellectual Disability Research, 67*(8), 701–719.

Bertapelli, F., Pitetti, K., Agiovlasitis, S., & Guerra-Junior, G. (2016). Overweight and obesity in children and adolescents with Down syndrome—Prevalence, determinants, consequences, and interventions: A literature review. *Research in Developmental Disabilities, 57*, 181–192.

Białek-Dratwa, A., Żur, S., Wilemska-Kucharzewska, K., Szczepańska, E., & Kowalski, O. (2022). Nutrition as prevention of diet-related diseases—A cross-sectional study among children and young adults with Down syndrome. *Children, 10*(1), 36.

Bittles, A., & Glasson, E. (2004). Clinical, social, and ethical implications of changing life expectancy in Down syndrome. *Developmental Medicine and Child Neurology, 46*(4), 282–286.

Bull, M. J., & Genetics Co. (2011). *Health supervision for children with Down syndrome* (pp. 393–406). American Academy of Pediatrics Elk Grove Village.

Bull, M. J., Trotter, T., Santoro, S. L., Christensen, C., Grout, R. W., & Co, G. (2022). Health supervision for children and adolescents with Down syndrome. *Pediatrics, 149*(5), e2022057010.

Cogulu, O., Ozkinay, F., Gunduz, C., Cankaya, T., Aydogdu, S., Ozgenc, F., et al. (2003). Celiac disease in children with Down syndrome: Importance of follow-up and serologic screening. *Pediatrics International, 45*(4), 395–399.

Coppedè, F. (2016). Risk factors for Down syndrome. *Archives of Toxicology, 90*(12), 2917–2929.

Dimopoulos, K., Constantine, A., Clift, P., Condliffe, R., Moledina, S., Jansen, K., et al. (2023). Cardiovascular complications of Down syndrome: Scoping review and expert consensus. *Circulation, 147*(5), 425–441.

Down Syndrome Australia. (2015). *Nutrition, weight management and physical fitness: Some basic considerations*. Down Syndrome Australia. https://www.downsyndrome.org.au/voice/wp-content/uploads/sites/4/2015/09/Nurtritionweightmanagementphysicalfitness.pdf

Down Syndrome Medical Interest Group (DSMIG). (2022). *Feeding and nutrition*. Down Syndrome Medical Interest Group (DSMIG). Retrieved January 7, 2022, from https://www.dsmig.org.uk/information-resources/by-topic/feeding-and-nutrition

Down's Syndrome Medical Interest Group (DSMIG). (2020). *Gastrointestinal conditions in adults*. Down's Syndrome UK (DSMIG). Retrieved October 25, 2020, from https://www.downs-syndrome.org.uk/wp-content/uploads/2020/06/Gastrointestinal-conditions-in-adults-Final-25th-Oct-DSMIG.pdf

Estigarribia, B. (2025). Language characteristics of individuals with Down syndrome. *Topics in Language Disorders, 29*, 112.

Ghosh, S., Feingold, E., & Dey, S. K. (2009). Etiology of Down syndrome: Evidence for consistent association among altered meiotic recombination, nondisjunction, and maternal age across populations. *American Journal of Medical Genetics Part A, 149*(7), 1415–1420.

Gruszka, J., & Włodarek, D. (2024). General dietary recommendations for people with Down syndrome. *Nutrients, 16*(16), 2656.

Hefti, E., & Blanco, J. G. (2017). Pharmacotherapeutic considerations for individuals with Down syndrome. *Pharmacotherapy: The Journal of Human Pharmacology and Drug Therapy, 37*(2), 214–220.

Illinois Department of Central Management Services / Be Well Illinois. (n.d.). *Down syndrome and nutrition*. Be Well Illinois / CMS Illinois. https://cms.illinois.gov/benefits/stateemployee/bewell/foodforthought/october23-down-syndrome-and-nutrition.html

Irish Nutrition & Dietetic Institute (INDI). (2023). *Nutrition and diet for children and adults with Down syndrome*. Retrieved May 2023, from https://www.indi.ie/diseases%2C-allergies-and-medical-conditions/disability/396-down-syndrome-and-nutrition.html

Lima, A. S., Cardoso, B. R., & Cozzolino, S. F. (2010). Nutritional status of zinc in children with Down syndrome. *Biological Trace Element Research, 133*(1), 20–28.

Luke, A., Sutton, M., Schoeller, D. A., & Roizen, N. J. (1996). Nutrient intake and obesity in prepubescent children with Down syndrome. *Journal of the American Dietetic Association, 96*(12), 1262–1267.

Lyon, P., Strippoli, V., Fang, B., & Cimmino, L. (2020). B vitamins and one-carbon metabolism: Implications in human health and disease. *Nutrients, 12*(9), 2867.

Morris, J., Mutton, D., & Alberman, E. (2005). Recurrences of free trisomy 21: Analysis of data from the national Down syndrome cytogenetic register. *Prenatal Diagnosis: Published in Affiliation With the International Society for Prenatal Diagnosis, 25*(12), 1120–1128.

National Center on Health PAaDN. (n.d.). *Nutrition considerations for individuals with Down syndrome*. NCHPAD. https://www.nchpad.org/resources/down-syndrome-and-nutrition

National Down Syndrome Society. (n.d.). *Nutrition and Down syndrome*. https://ndss.org/resources/nutrition

Nordstrøm, M., Retterstøl, K., Hope, S., & Kolset, S. O. (2020). Nutritional challenges in children and adolescents with Down syndrome. *The Lancet Child & Adolescent Health, 4*(6), 455–464.

Palumbo, M. L., & McDougle, C. J. (2018). Pharmacotherapy of Down syndrome. *Expert Opinion on Pharmacotherapy, 19*(17), 1875–1889.

Ravel, A., Mircher, C., Rebillat, A.-S., Cieuta-Walti, C., & Megarbane, A. (2020). Feeding problems and gastrointestinal diseases in Down syndrome. *Archives de Pédiatrie, 27*(1), 53–60.

Rogers, J.C., Elizabeth, & Howells, A. (n.d.). *Helping constipation—Preventing & improving management of constipation*. https://www.downsyndromeuk.co.uk/docs/All%20things%20toileting/12839%20P4S%20Helping%20Constipation-Preventing%20%26%20improving%20management.pdf

Roizen, N. J., & Patterson, D. (2003). Down's syndrome. *The Lancet, 361*(9365), 1281–1289.

Romano, C., Van Wynckel, M., Hulst, J., Broekaert, I., Bronsky, J., Dall'Oglio, L., et al. (2017). European society for paediatric gastroenterology, hepatology and nutrition guidelines for the evaluation and treatment of gastrointestinal and nutritional complications in children with neurological impairment. *Journal of Pediatric Gastroenterology and Nutrition, 65*(2), 242–264.

Roper, R. J., & Reeves, R. H. (2006). Understanding the basis for Down syndrome phenotypes. *PLoS Genetics, 2*(3), e50.

Rueda Revilla, N., & Martínez-Cué, C. (2020). Antioxidants in Down syndrome: From preclinical studies to clinical trials. *Antioxidants, 9*(8), 692.

Saghazadeh, A., Mahmoudi, M., Dehghani Ashkezari, A., Oliaie Rezaie, N., & Rezaei, N. (2017). Systematic review and meta-analysis shows a specific micronutrient profile in people with Down syndrome: Lower blood calcium, selenium and zinc, higher red blood cell copper and zinc, and higher salivary calcium and sodium. *PLoS One, 12*(4), e0175437.

Shahidi, F., & Ambigaipalan, P. (2018). Omega-3 polyunsaturated fatty acids and their health benefits. *Annual Review of Food Science and Technology, 9*(1), 345–381.

Sherman, S. L., Allen, E. G., Bean, L. H., & Freeman, S. B. (2007). Epidemiology of Down syndrome. *Mental Retardation and Developmental Disabilities Research Reviews, 13*(3), 221–227.

Shirode, P. S., Parekh, A. D., Patel, V. V., Vala, J., Jaimalani, A. M., Vora, N. M., et al. (2023). Early detection of subclinical atherosclerosis: Hyperhomocysteinemia as a promising marker in adolescents with vitamin B deficiency. *Cureus, 15*(7), e41571.

Ulrich, D. A., Burghardt, A. R., Lloyd, M., Tiernan, C., & Hornyak, J. E. (2011). Physical activity benefits of learning to ride a two-wheel bicycle for children with Down syndrome: A randomized trial. *Physical Therapy, 91*(10), 1463–1477.

Vraneković, J., Slivšek, G., & Majstorović, D. (2020). Methyltetrahydrofolate-homocysteine methyltransferase reductase gene and congenital heart defects in Down syndrome. *Genetics&Applications, 4*(1), 12–17.

Weijerman, M. E., & De Winter, J. P. (2010). Clinical practice: The care of children with Down syndrome. *European Journal of Pediatrics, 169*(12), 1445–1452.

Whooten, R., Schmitt, J., & Schwartz, A. (2018). Endocrine manifestations of Down syndrome. *Current Opinion in Endocrinology, Diabetes and Obesity, 25*(1), 61–66.

Żur, S., Sokal, A., Staśkiewicz-Bartecka, W., Kiciak, A., Grajek, M., Krupa-Kotara, K., et al. (2025). Nutrition for children with Down syndrome—Current knowledge, challenges, and clinical recommendations—A narrative review. *Healthcare, 13*, 2222. MDPI.

Chapter 4
Autism Spectrum Disorder

Abstract

- Autism Spectrum Disorder (ASD) is introduced as a neurodevelopmental disability disorder within the broader category of pervasive developmental disorders (PDD) and typically becomes evident by the age of three, presenting with persistent difficulties in communication, social interaction, and behavior, with a global prevalence of 1–3% and higher occurrence among boys.
- The etiology of ASD is described as multifactorial, combining genetic predisposition, prenatal and perinatal complications, nutritional and metabolic influences, immune dysfunction, and environmental exposures such as pollutants, heavy metals, and maternal medication use during pregnancy.
- The nutritional management in ASD is challenging because cognitive rigidity, sensory sensitivities, and food selectivity often lead to feeding difficulties, gastrointestinal problems, obesity, and inadequate nutrient intake, requiring tailored interventions.
- The nutrition-related challenges in ASD include gastrointestinal complications like constipation and diarrhea, a higher risk of obesity, and deficiencies in key vitamins (A, D, E, B12, folate), minerals (iron, zinc, selenium, magnesium), and fatty acids, making supplementation frequently necessary.
- The medical nutrition therapy involves approaches such as gluten-free/casein-free diets, antioxidant-rich diets, and ketogenic diets, though evidence for consistent benefit is limited, so individualized and supervised planning is recommended.
- Although there is no cure for ASD and no specific medication to treat the condition directly, pharmacological interventions are widely used to manage comorbid symptoms such as depression, seizures, insomnia, and attention difficulties, and highlights the importance of monitoring food–drug interactions, as medications like antipsychotics, antidepressants, stimulants, and anticonvulsants may have significant interactions with alcohol, caffeine, grapefruit juice, or herbal products.

M. H. Rouhani et al., *The Healing Plate*, SpringerBriefs in Modern Perspectives on Disability Research, https://doi.org/10.1007/978-981-95-8150-4_4

Keywords Autism spectrum disorder (ASD) · Neurodevelopmental disorders · Nutrition · Feeding difficulties · Gastrointestinal complications · Micronutrients · Obesity · Dietary interventions · Supplementation · Food–drug interactions

4.1 Definition and Epidemiology

Autism Spectrum Disorder (ASD) is a neurodevelopmental disability within the broader category of pervasive developmental disorders (PDD), typically evident by the age of three. It is characterized by persistent challenges in communication, social interaction, and behavior. While the presentation varies widely, individuals with ASD may display differences in speech—from advanced conversational skills to complete absence of verbal communication—and in functional abilities, ranging from independent living to requiring substantial daily support (Association AP, 2013; Centers for Disease Control and Prevention, 2025a; World Health Organization, 2023).

ASD affects individuals across all racial, ethnic, and socioeconomic groups, with a global prevalence of approximately 1–3% in children. Recent estimates from the U.S. Centers for Disease Control and Prevention (CDC) report a prevalence of 1 in 31 children aged 8 years (Centers for Disease Control and Prevention, 2025b).

4.2 Etiology

Several factors are associated with an increased risk of ASD, including male sex, a positive family history, coexisting genetic or neurological conditions such as *Fragile X syndrome*, *Tuberous sclerosis*, or *Rett syndrome*, preterm birth before 26 weeks of gestation, and advanced maternal or paternal age at conception. While these factors influence susceptibility, they do not represent definitive causes of the disorder.

Although the precise etiology of ASD remains elusive, current research points to a multifactorial origin involving genetic predisposition in combination with environmental, nutritional, metabolic, immunological, and neurobiological influences. Environmental risk factors under investigation include exposure to air pollutants, heavy metals such as lead, chemically treated foods, and hormonal additives in meat. Nutritional elements of interest encompass the role of neurotransmitters, essential fatty acids, antioxidant nutrients (vitamins A, C, and E, selenium), and minerals such as zinc, calcium, and magnesium, alongside dietary approaches like mercury-free or allergen-elimination regimens. Additional factors linked to increased risk include advanced parental age—both paternal and maternal—and maternal use of certain medications during pregnancy (Augustyn, 2024; Boddaert et al., 2009; Centers for Disease Control and Prevention, 2025a; Lai et al., 2014; Sandin et al., 2012).

4.3 Nutritional Management

Core ASD characteristics such as cognitive rigidity, resistance to change, and sensory processing difficulties frequently lead to feeding problems. A summary of the most frequently reported issues is provided in Box 4.1.

Box 4.1 Common Nutrition and Eating-Related Issues in Children with Autism Spectrum Disorder

- Limited dietary variety and refusal to try new foods.
- Inadequate intake of energy/fiber/calcium/vitamin D/iron/other nutrient(s).
- Underweight or overweight/obesity.
- Short attention span during meals.
- Heightened sensory sensitivities to food textures, colors, tastes, or temperatures.
- Pica—consumption of non-food items.
- Compulsive eating or drinking behaviors.
- Mouth packing (holding excessive amounts of food in the mouth).
- Vomiting and exaggerated gag reflex.
- Gastrointestinal disturbances resembling celiac disease.

Intolerances to gluten and casein proteins have been proposed to contribute to intestinal inflammation and the production of brain opioids, although current scientific evidence remains limited. Nevertheless, gluten-free and casein-free diets have become popular complementary and alternative therapies among caregivers of children with ASD. No single dietary intervention is universally effective for all individuals with ASD. Therefore, medical nutrition therapy should be tailored to each child and integrated alongside behavioral management, speech and occupational therapies, and counseling (Al-Beltagi, 2024; Whiteley et al., 2012).

4.3.1 Nutrition-Related Challenges

Ensuring sufficient nutritional intake represents a significant challenge for children with ASD. Research indicates that nearly 90% of affected children experience feeding-related anxiety (Cekici & Sanlier, 2019). Gastrointestinal (GI) complications—such as constipation, diarrhea, and steatorrhea—along with food allergies, metabolic abnormalities, and feeding disorders, frequently hinder adequate nutrient absorption and intake in this population. Supplementation with multivitamins and minerals has been associated with improvements in autism-related symptoms, potentially through their role in alleviating GI disturbances commonly observed in children with ASD (Berry et al., 2015; Holingue et al., 2018).

Gastrointestinal Complications

GI disorders are frequently observed in children with ASD. A meta-analysis has demonstrated that GI complaints in this population are significantly associated with a higher risk of constipation, diarrhea, and abdominal pain. Food selectivity (FS) in children with ASD has been strongly associated with a higher prevalence of gastrointestinal GI symptoms, particularly constipation and diarrhea. These children often show a preference for foods rich in simple carbohydrates, such as sweets, while avoiding fiber-rich fruits and vegetables, a pattern that may exacerbate GI disturbances (Berry et al., 2015; Chakraborty et al., 2021; McElhanon et al., 2014; Sun et al., 2013).

Children with ASD exhibit a less diverse gut microbiota compared to typically developing peers. Specifically, *Bifidobacterium* and *Firmicutes* are often found at reduced levels, whereas *Clostridium*, *Bacteroidetes*, and *Sarcina* are present in higher abundance (Kilinç & Söğüt, 2018). A systematic review indicated that specific probiotics and dietary interventions may support the restoration of healthy gut microbiota and enhance gastrointestinal (GI) health (Al-Ayadhi et al., 2021).

Weight Management

Weight gain and obesity are more prevalent among children with ASD compared to typically developing peers. This increased risk may result from atypical eating patterns, dietary rigidity, hypersensitivity to sensory characteristics of food, sedentary lifestyle, comorbid conditions, and the use of certain medications. Additional contributing factors include reduced gut microbiota diversity, hormonal dysregulation, and maternal metabolic disturbances (Buro et al., 2022; Sammels et al., 2022).

Nutritional Deficiencies

Although the overall nutrient requirements of children with ASD are comparable to those of typically developing children, factors such as food selectivity, gastrointestinal disturbances, and restrictive eating behaviors frequently result in inadequate micronutrient intake. This insufficiency may exacerbate both core and associated symptoms of autism. Several studies have reported that children with ASD often exhibit lower intake levels of key micronutrients, including magnesium, selenium, vitamins A, D, and E, folate, and iron (Chakraborty et al., 2021; Hyman et al., 2012; Nogueira-de-Almeida et al., 2025; Peretti et al., 2019).

Children with ASD frequently experience feeding difficulties, prompting caregivers to use dietary supplements to support nutritional adequacy. While multivitamin and mineral formulations are commonly administered, they often fail to provide sufficient amounts of certain micronutrients, such as choline and potassium, which are frequently deficient in this population. The most prevalent nutritional insufficiencies involve vitamins, minerals, and essential fatty acids. Specifically, reduced intake and serum levels of pantothenic acid, folate, biotin, vitamin B12, vitamin D,

Table 4.1 Commonly used supplements in autism spectrum disorder with potential beneficial effects on symptoms

- Water-soluble vitamins supplements plus Vitamin D
- Omega-3 fatty acids
- Mineral supplements including magnesium, zinc, and selenium
- Probiotics
- Melatonin, glutathione, and L-carnitine

and vitamin E have been documented. Moreover, impairments in key metabolic pathways, including cellular methylation and glutathione-dependent antioxidant defenses, have been reported. Supplementation with vitamin B12 is hypothesized to enhance methylation processes and antioxidant capacity, while antioxidants such as vitamins C and E are commonly utilized to counteract elevated oxidative stress in children with ASD (Al-Beltagi, 2024; Gogou & Kolios, 2017; Jayashree et al., 2024; Li et al., 2018; Nogueira-de-Almeida et al., 2025; Peretti et al., 2019; Sathe et al., 2017). Common supplements used in ASD are presented in Table 4.1.

4.3.2 Medical Nutrition Therapy

Various dietary interventions, including antioxidant-rich diets, gluten-free (GF)/casein-free (CF) diets, and ketogenic diets, have been associated with improvements in ASD-related symptoms. Among these, the GF/CF diet is the most widely implemented; although most studies have not demonstrated significant measurable benefits, caregivers frequently report subtle behavioral improvements (Sathe et al., 2017). It is proposed that the GF/CF diet, or the related specific carbohydrate diet (SCD), may benefit a subset of children by targeting underlying gastrointestinal or immune dysfunctions commonly present in ASD, rather than directly addressing core autism features (Garcia et al., 2017). Other dietary strategies, such as elimination diets and additive-free diets, have shown limited potential for symptom improvement, yet in some cases may result in adverse effects, including inadequate or excessive nutrient intake. Overall, current evidence remains insufficient to support the routine use of these dietary interventions as standard therapeutic strategies for ASD (Alam et al., 2023; Al-Beltagi, 2024; Cekici & Sanlier, 2019; Karhu et al., 2020; Leader et al., 2022; Ozler & Sanlier, 2025; Sathe et al., 2017).

4.4 Food–Drug Interaction

Although there is no cure for ASD and no specific medication to treat the condition directly, pharmacological interventions can be useful in managing related symptoms such as depression, seizures, insomnia, and difficulty concentrating. The

Table 4.2 summarizes these drug categories, along with their common examples, and notable food–drug interaction (Angelakou, n.d.; Applied Behavior Analysis EDU, 2017; LeClerc & Easley, 2015; Siegel & Erickson, 2017).

Table 4.2 Commonly Prescribed Medications for Autism Spectrum Disorder and Their Food–Drug Interactions

Drug	Trade Name	Food–Drug Interaction
Antipsychotics		
Risperidone	Risperdal	**Side effects:** Increased appetite, **Avoid:** Not be mixed with tea or cola, avoid or limit the use of alcohol
Aripiprazole	Abilify	**Avoid:** Alcohol
Antidepressants		
Fluoxetine (*SSRI*)	Prozac	**Side effects:** Anorexia, hypokalemia **Avoid:** Alcohol
Fluvoxamine (*SSRI*)	Luvox	**Avoid:** Alcohol
Sertraline (*SSRI*)	Zoloft	**Avoid:** Alcohol, St John's wort, and grapefruit or grapefruit juice
Citalopram (*SSRI*)	Celexa	**Avoid:** St John's wort and alcohol
Venlafaxine (SNRI)	Effexor	**Avoid:** Alcohol
Clomipramine (TCA)	Anafranil	**Side effects:** Increased appetite, **Avoid:** Grapefruit, grapefruit juice, cranberry juice, alcohol
Stimulants		
Methylphenidate	Ritalin	**Side effects:** Anorexia **Avoid:** Caffeine and alcohol
Mixed amphetamine salts	Adderall	**Side effects:** Anorexia **Avoid:** Alcohol
Anticonvulsants		
Valproic acid	Depakote	**Side effects:** Increased appetite, causes nutrient depletions (zinc—selenium—folic acid—vitamin B3 deficiencies) **Avoid:** Alcohol
Phenytoin	Dilantin	**Side effects:** Causes nutrient depletions (hypocalcemia, folic acid—vitamin B1—vitamin B12—vitamin K deficiencies), increases use of vitamin D in the body **Avoid:** Alcohol
Clonazepam	Klonopin	**Avoid:** Alcohol
Carbamazepine	Tegretol	**Side effects:** Weight gain and causes nutrient depletions (folic acid, biotin, and vitamin D) **Avoid:** St John's wort, grapefruit juice, pomegranate juice, and alcohol
Other		
Naltrexone	Revia	**Side effects:** Anorexia **Avoid:** Alcohol
Alprazolam	Xanax	**Side effects:** Increased appetite **Avoid:** Grapefruit, grapefruit juice, and alcohol

Acknowledgments The authors confirm that the content, analysis, and conclusions of this manuscript are their own work. AI-based tools were used solely to assist in improving the clarity and correctness of the English language.

References

Alam, S., Westmark, C. J., & McCullagh, E. A. (2023). Diet in treatment of autism spectrum disorders. *Frontiers in Neuroscience, 16*, 1031016.

Al-Ayadhi, L., Zayed, N., Bhat, R. S., Moubayed, N. M., Al-Muammar, M. N., & El-Ansary, A. (2021). The use of biomarkers associated with leaky gut as a diagnostic tool for early intervention in autism spectrum disorder: A systematic review. *Gut Pathogens, 13*(1), 54.

Al-Beltagi, M. (2024). Nutritional management and autism spectrum disorder: A systematic review. *World Journal of Clinical Pediatrics, 13*(4), 99649.

Angelakou, I. A.. (n.d.). *Food-drug interactions and their impact on the pharmacotherapy*.

Applied Behavior Analysis EDU. (2017). *What drugs are used for treating autism?* Applied Behavior Analysis EDU. https://www.appliedbehavioranalysisedu.org/what-drugs-are-used-for-treating-autism

Association AP. (2013). *Autism spectrum disorder. Diagnostic and statistical manual of mental disorders*, 5.

Augustyn, M. (2024). *Autism spectrum disorder (ASD) in children and adolescents: Terminology, epidemiology, and pathogenesis*. UptoDate. Retrieved July 29, 2024.

Berry, R. C., Novak, P., Withrow, N., Schmidt, B., Rarback, S., Feucht, S., et al. (2015). Nutrition management of gastrointestinal symptoms in children with autism spectrum disorder: Guideline from an expert panel. *Journal of the Academy of Nutrition and Dietetics, 115*(12), 1919–1927.

Boddaert, N., Zilbovicius, M., Philipe, A., Robel, L., Bourgeois, M., Barthélemy, C., et al. (2009). MRI findings in 77 children with non-syndromic autistic disorder. *PLoS One, 4*(2), e4415.

Buro, A. W., Salinas-Miranda, A., Marshall, J., Gray, H. L., & Kirby, R. S. (2022). Obesity and co-occurring conditions among adolescents with autism spectrum disorder: The national survey of children's health 2017–2018. *Research in Autism Spectrum Disorders, 92*, 101927.

Cekici, H., & Sanlier, N. (2019). Current nutritional approaches in managing autism spectrum disorder: A review. *Nutritional Neuroscience, 22*(3), 145–155.

Centers for Disease Control and Prevention. (2025a). *Autism spectrum disorder (ASD)*. U.S. Department of Health & Human Services. Retrieved May 2025, from https://www.cdc.gov/autism/index.html

Centers for Disease Control and Prevention. (2025b). *Data and statistics on autism spectrum disorder*. Centers for Disease Control and Prevention. https://www.cdc.gov/autism/data-research/index.html

Chakraborty, P., Carpenter, K. L., Major, S., Deaver, M., Vermeer, S., Herold, B., et al. (2021). Gastrointestinal problems are associated with increased repetitive behaviors but not social communication difficulties in young children with autism spectrum disorders. *Autism, 25*(2), 405–415.

Garcia, M. J., McPherson, P., Patel, S. Y., & Burns, C. O. (2017). Diet and supplementation targeted for autism spectrum disorder. In *Handbook of treatments for autism spectrum disorder* (pp. 397–425). Springer.

Gogou, M., & Kolios, G. (2017). The effect of dietary supplements on clinical aspects of autism spectrum disorder: A systematic review of the literature. *Brain and Development, 39*(8), 656–664.

Holingue, C., Newill, C., Lee, L. C., Pasricha, P. J., & Daniele, F. M. (2018). Gastrointestinal symptoms in autism spectrum disorder: A review of the literature on ascertainment and prevalence. *Autism Research, 11*(1), 24–36.

Hyman, S. L., Stewart, P. A., Schmidt, B., Cain, U., Lemcke, N., Foley, J. T., et al. (2012). Nutrient intake from food in children with autism. *Pediatrics, 130*(Supplement_2), S145–SS53.

Jayashree, R., Gayathri, G., & Udayakumar, N. (2024). Nutritional supplements in autism spectrum disorder: A scoping review. *International Journal of Nutrition, Pharmacology, Neurological Diseases, 14*(2), 153–156.

Karhu, E., Zukerman, R., Eshraghi, R. S., Mittal, J., Deth, R. C., Castejon, A. M., et al. (2020). Nutritional interventions for autism spectrum disorder. *Nutrition Reviews, 78*(7), 515–531.

Kilinç, G. E., & Söğüt, M. Ü. (2018). Mikrobiyotaya güncel bir yaklaşım: otizm ve mikrobiyota. *Turkiye Klinikleri Journal of Health Sciences, 3*(1), 88–94.

Lai, M.-C., Lombardo, M. V., & Baron-Cohen, S. (2014). Autism. *Lancet, 383*(9920), 896–910.

Leader, G., Abberton, C., Cunningham, S., Gilmartin, K., Grudzien, M., Higgins, E., et al. (2022). Gastrointestinal symptoms in autism spectrum disorder: A systematic review. *Nutrients, 14*(7), 1471.

LeClerc, S., & Easley, D. (2015). Pharmacological therapies for autism spectrum disorder: A review. *P t., 40*(6), 389–397.

Li, Y.-J., Li, Y.-M., & Xiang, D.-X. (2018). Supplement intervention associated with nutritional deficiencies in autism spectrum disorders: A systematic review. *European Journal of Nutrition, 57*(7), 2571–2582.

McElhanon, B. O., McCracken, C., Karpen, S., & Sharp, W. G. (2014). Gastrointestinal symptoms in autism spectrum disorder: A meta-analysis. *Pediatrics, 133*(5), 872–883.

Nogueira-de-Almeida, C. A., de Araújo, L. A., da V. Ued, F., Contini, A. A., Nogueira-de-Almeida, M. E., Martinez, E. Z., et al. (2025). Nutritional factors and therapeutic interventions in autism spectrum disorder: A narrative review. *Children, 12*(2), 202.

Ozler, E., & Sanlier, N. (2025). Nutritional approaches in autism spectrum disorder: A scoping review. *Current Nutrition Reports, 14*(1), 61.

Peretti, S., Mariano, M., Mazzocchetti, C., Mazza, M., Pino, M., Verrotti Di Pianella, A., et al. (2019). Diet: The keystone of autism spectrum disorder? *Nutritional Neuroscience, 22*(12), 825–839.

Sammels, O., Karjalainen, L., Dahlgren, J., & Wentz, E. (2022). Autism spectrum disorder and obesity in children: A systematic review and meta-analysis. *Obesity Facts, 15*(3), 305–320.

Sandin, S., Hultman, C. M., Kolevzon, A., Gross, R., MacCabe, J. H., & Reichenberg, A. (2012). Advancing maternal age is associated with increasing risk for autism: A review and meta-analysis. *Journal of the American Academy of Child & Adolescent Psychiatry, 51*(5), 477–86.e1.

Sathe, N., Andrews, J. C., McPheeters, M. L., & Warren, Z. E. (2017). Nutritional and dietary interventions for autism spectrum disorder: A systematic review. *Pediatrics, 139*(6), e20170346.

Siegel, M., & Erickson, C. (2017) *Autism spectrum disorder: Parents' medication guide*. American Academy of Child and Adolescent Psychiatry. https://www.aacap.org/App_Themes/AACAP/Docs/resource_centers/autism/Autism_Spectrum_Disorder_Parents_Medication_Guide.pdf

Sun, C., Xia, W., Zhao, Y., Li, N., Zhao, D., & Wu, L. (2013). Nutritional status survey of children with autism and typically developing children aged 4–6 years in Heilongjiang province. *China. Journal of Nutritional Science, 2*, e16.

Whiteley, P., Shattock, P., Knivsberg, A. M., Seim, A., Reichelt, K. L., Todd, L., et al. (2012). Gluten—And casein-free dietary intervention for autism spectrum conditions. *Frontiers in Human Neuroscience, 6*, 344.

World Health Organization. (2023). *Autism spectrum disorders*. World Health Organization. https://www.who.int/news-room/fact-sheets/detail/autism-spectrum-disorders

Chapter 5
Cerebral Palsy

Abstract

- Cerebral Palsy (CP) is a lifelong neurodevelopmental disability disorder characterized by motor impairments affecting muscle tone, posture, and movement, resulting from brain injury during fetal or infant development.
- Epidemiology indicates a prevalence of about 2 per 1000 live births in the United States, while some regions report 3–4 per 1000. The birth prevalence is significantly higher in low- and middle-income countries than in high-income countries, and most diagnoses occur between 9 and 12 months of age.
- Clinical presentation includes delays in motor milestones (sitting, walking), abnormal muscle tone (stiffness or floppiness), feeding/swallowing problems, drooling, constipation, reflux, bladder dysfunction, and later-life osteoporosis.
- Etiology is multifactorial, involving prenatal, perinatal, and genetic risk factors such as maternal infections, prematurity, low birth weight, and genetic mutations.
- Nutrition-related challenges include dysphagia, feeding difficulties, malnutrition, GI complications, and risk of both undernutrition and overweight/obesity.
- Bone health concerns involve vitamin D and calcium deficiency, low bone density, and fracture risk, requiring supplementation and, in severe cases, bisphosphonate therapy.
- Medical nutrition therapy focuses on individualized energy, protein, micronutrient, and fluid needs, with early interventions and monitoring.
- Enteral tube feeding is indicated when oral intake is insufficient, using appropriate formulas to match energy needs.
- Food–drug interactions are important, as common medications may affect appetite, nutrient absorption, and weight, requiring careful dietary and clinical management.

Keywords Cerebral palsy (CP) · Neurodevelopmental disorders · Motor impairments · Feeding difficulties · Dysphagia · Malnutrition · Bone health · Micronutrients · Enteral nutrition · Food–drug interactions

M. H. Rouhani et al., *The Healing Plate*, SpringerBriefs in Modern Perspectives on Disability Research, https://doi.org/10.1007/978-981-95-8150-4_5

5.1 Definition and Epidemiology

Cerebral palsy (CP) refers to a group of disorders that cause lifelong motor impairments, affecting muscle tone, posture, and movement. These impairments result from damage to the brain during its development in the fetus or infant (Rosenbaum et al., 2007). The prevalence of CP in the United States is estimated at about 2 cases per 1000 live births, whereas in some regions worldwide, the rate may be higher, approximately 3 to 4 cases per 1000 live births. The birth prevalence of CP is significantly higher in low- and middle-income countries compared to high-income ones (Jahan et al., 2021; McIntyre et al., 2022; Oskoui et al., 2013; Van Naarden et al., 2016).

CP primarily presents with difficulties in movement, coordination, and overall motor development. Children may show delays in achieving milestones, such as sitting by 8 months or walking by 18 months, and often exhibit abnormal muscle tone, either excessive stiffness or unusual floppiness. In addition to motor problems, children with CP may experience feeding and swallowing difficulties, drooling, constipation, gastroesophageal reflux, and bladder dysfunction. In addition, decreased bone mineral density and the development of osteoporosis may manifest in later adulthood (NHS, 2023; NINDS, 2025).

CP is classified into four main types according to neurological manifestations, including spastic, dyskinetic, ataxic, and mixed CP. CP is most commonly diagnosed between 9 and 12 months of age. In addition, the mobility and gross motor abilities of individuals with CP are classified into five distinct levels through the Gross Motor Function Classification System (GMFCS), which provides a standardized framework for describing motor function (Cerebral Palsy Alliance Research Foundation, n.d.; NHS, 2023). The details of this classification are presented in the Box 5.1.

Box 5.1 Gross Motor Function Classification System (GMFCS)

Level I—Walks without limitations.

Walks without limitations indoors or outdoors, climbs stairs without hand support, can run and jump, with slight reductions in speed, balance, and coordination.

Level II—Walking with Limitations.

Walks indoors and outdoors and climbs stairs using a railing; has difficulty on uneven terrain, inclines, or in crowds; minimal running or jumping.

Level III—Walks using a hand-held mobility device.

Uses hand-held mobility aids on level surfaces; may climb stairs with support; can propel a manual wheelchair short distance, requiring assistance for longer or uneven surfaces.

Level IV—Self-mobility with limitations, may use powered mobility.
Walking severely limited even with aids; primarily uses a wheelchair (manual or powered); may participate in supported standing or transfers.
Level V—Transported in a manual wheelchair.
Severe motor impairments restrict voluntary movement and postural control; independent sitting, standing, and walking are not possible; may use powered mobility.

- Feeding Capabilities:

  Oral feeding without a tube
  Feeding via tube

5.2 Etiology

The etiology of CP is complex and often multifactorial, involving a wide range of factors that may negatively affect the developing fetal or neonatal brain. Several potentially modifiable prenatal influences have been linked to an increased risk of CP, including heavy maternal alcohol intake, cigarette smoking, and obesity. Babies born with a low birth weight, typically under 3.3 pounds (1.5 kilograms), are also more vulnerable (Cleveland Clinic, 2025; Korzeniewski et al., 2018; Potcovaru et al., 2022).

Findings from a large case-control study highlighted that the strongest independent predictors of CP were a low 5-min Apgar score, intrauterine infection, and maternal drug use (Rouabhi et al., 2023). Additional contributors included maternal tobacco exposure, prolonged rupture of membranes, diabetes, preeclampsia, preterm birth, low birth weight, male sex, and a history of previous miscarriages. Beyond environmental and perinatal factors, genetic contributions have also been recognized, which studies suggesting that genetic abnormalities may account for approximately 8% to over 30% of CP cases (Fahey et al., 2017; MacLennan et al., 2015; McMichael et al., 2015; Moreno-De-Luca et al., 2012; Moreno-De-Luca et al., 2021; Schaefer, 2008).

Preventive strategies have been explored, particularly in high-risk pregnancies. Clinical trials provide evidence that antenatal administration of magnesium sulfate to women at risk of preterm delivery can lower both the incidence and severity of CP without increasing mortality (Korzeniewski et al., 2018).

5.3 Nutritional Management

5.3.1 Nutrition-Related Challenges

Children with CP are particularly vulnerable to feeding difficulties and malnutrition due to multiple nutrition-related factors. Low muscle tone and weakness in the muscles of the face, tongue, jaw, and throat can interfere with chewing and make swallowing unsafe or inefficient. In addition, impaired motor coordination and reduced strength in the arms and hands often hinder self-feeding skills, further limiting adequate intake. Frequent hospitalizations and recurrent infections associated with CP may also increase metabolic demands, thereby intensifying the need for nutritional support. Moreover, many children with CP experience gastrointestinal (GI) complications such as constipation and gastroesophageal reflux disease, which can further compromise comfort during meals and reduce overall nutritional adequacy. This point should be taken into account that children with CP are not only at risk of undernutrition but may also experience overweight or obesity. This can occur when dietary choices prioritize foods that are palatable and easy to consume rather than nutritionally balanced. Limited physical activity, often resulting from motor impairments, further contributes to the risk of excessive weight gain in these children. These points highlight the dual burden of malnutrition in children with CP, where both undernutrition and overnutrition can significantly affect overall health and quality of life (Center BI, 2023).

Dysphagia

Dysphagia, or difficulty in swallowing, is one of the most significant contributors to nutritional problems in CP children. It interferes not only with safe and efficient food intake but also increases the risk of aspiration, choking, and respiratory complications. Dysphagia is particularly common in children with moderate to severe motor impairment.

Management of dysphagia involves strategies such as modifying food texture and consistency (e.g., softening, thickening, or thinning food and liquids as required), offering smaller and more frequent meals, and emphasizing thorough chewing. Therapeutic interventions, including muscle exercises guided by physical therapists or speech-language pathologists, can support safer and more effective swallowing. In severe cases, alternative feeding methods, such as feeding tube, may be required to ensure adequate nutrition and minimize health risks (Benfer et al., 2017; Edvinsson & Lundqvist, 2016; Erlichman, 1989; Graham et al., 2019; Kim et al., 2013; Yi et al., 2019).

Gastrointestinal Complications

Children with CP are at heightened risk of GI complications, which can significantly affect their nutritional status and overall quality of life. Common digestive issues include abdominal discomfort, vomiting, bloating, and particularly constipation, which may present as either acute or chronic and, in some cases, signal a more serious underlying disorder. Several factors contribute to these complications, including impaired feeding ability, abnormal body positioning, reduced mobility, muscle spasms, swallowing difficulties, and excessive drooling. Furthermore, feeding and digestion in children with CP may be accompanied by systemic changes such as fluctuations in breathing, heart rate, blood pressure, and mood.

Warning signs that warrant evaluation by a medical team include constipation, incontinence, feeding refusal or inability to feed, swallowing or sucking difficulties, unexplained weight loss or gain, recurrent vomiting, unusual fatigue, and choking or aspiration episodes. Early recognition of these symptoms is critical to prevent further nutritional deterioration.

Management of GI issues often involves referral to a gastroenterologist, who can develop individualized treatment plans following comprehensive evaluation. Interventions may include dietary modifications, the use of probiotics, or medications such as antispasmodics for bowel regulation. In some cases, referral to specialists in feeding and swallowing therapy is necessary to improve oral intake. Additionally, eliminating foods and beverages that trigger adverse reactions is a simple but effective strategy for reducing symptoms and enhancing nutritional well-being (Del Giudice et al., 1999; Erkin et al., 2010; Kuperminc & Stevenson, 2008; Rouster et al., 2016; Trivić & Hojsak, 2019).

Bone Health Problems

Adequate nutrition plays a fundamental role in bone mineralization in children with CP. However, bone health in these patients is influenced by multiple additional factors, including reduced mobility, history of fractures, low weight-for-age, and age-related decline in bone density. Among nutritional contributors, deficiencies in vitamin D and calcium are particularly important, with nearly half of children with CP showing vitamin D insufficiency and about one-third presenting with deficiency. Limited sun exposure, poor oral intake, feeding difficulties, reliance on formula feeding, and malnutrition are common contributing factors. Furthermore, the use of certain medications such as carbamazepine, phenytoin, and proton pump inhibitors can impair the absorption of vitamin D, calcium, and magnesium, further compromising bone health.

Management of these deficiencies involves ensuring adequate intake of calories, protein, and micronutrients (including zinc, magnesium, and phosphorus) to prevent malnutrition and preserve muscle and bone mass. Vitamin D supplementation is routinely recommended, and in cases of severe osteopenia, bisphosphonate therapy may be considered as part of a comprehensive treatment plan (Alenazi, 2022; Carman et al., 2022; Houlihan, 2014; Jesus & Stevenson, 2020; Junges et al., 2020; Le Roy et al., 2021; Modlesky & Zhang, 2020; Mus-Peters et al., 2019).

5.3.2 *Medical Nutrition Therapy*

Individualized dietary plans are developed with careful consideration of multiple factors, including the child's medical condition, environment, cultural background, food allergies or intolerances, and body composition measurements. A nutrition therapist also provides education and guidance to parents and caregivers, enabling them to meet the child's dietary needs both at home and in school settings.

Ongoing monitoring and assessment are critical to ensure that nutritional goals are achieved, appropriate supplements are provided when necessary, and feeding challenges are effectively addressed. Ultimately, medical nutrition therapy not only prevents malnutrition but also contributes to improved quality of life and overall health outcomes in children with CP.

Nutritional intervention should be initiated as early as possible once at-risk children are identified (Campanozzi & Staiano, 2010; Motil, 1994). Indications according to North American Society for Pediatric Gastroenterology, Hepatology and Nutrition (NASPGHAN) are presented in Box 5.2.

Box 5.2 Clinical Guideline to Initiate Nutritional Intervention in Children with Cerebral Palsy According to NASPGHAN

- Oral motor feeding difficulties with concurrent undernutrition (weight-for-height < 80% of expected; BMI <5th percentile).
- Growth failure (height-for-age < 90% of expected).
- Overweight (BMI >95th percentile).
- Individual nutrient deficiencies.

Estimation of Energy and Protein Requirements

Individualized assessment is essential, as energy requirements differ based on mobility, muscle tone, activity level, feeding difficulties, and the severity of disability. Children who are able to walk typically require energy amounts similar to their healthy peers, whereas those who rely on a wheelchair often need only 60–70% of that energy. The total energy expenditure to resting energy expenditure ratio in children with CP is approximately 1.5–1.6 in those with normal activity levels but may decrease to around 1.1 in children with quadriplegic CP. Adjustment of caloric intake should, therefore, be based not only on growth parameters but also on motor subtype and functional capacity. Recommended estimates include approximately 11 kcal/cm body length for spastic children or those with severely restricted mobility (ages 5–11 years), 14 kcal/cm for moderately active children in the same age group, and 45 kcal/kg for athetoid patients over 18 years of age. For clinical practice, ESPGHAN suggests the use of the

Schofield equation to estimate basal energy needs and Andrew et al. equation to estimate total energy requirements as starting points, while emphasizing the importance of ongoing monitoring and adjustment of dietary interventions. Although indirect calorimetry remains the gold standard for determining energy expenditure, it is rarely feasible in routine clinical settings. Consequently, most clinicians rely on the Dietary Reference Intakes (DRIs) and individualize nutritional prescriptions accordingly (Culley & Middleton TO, 1969; European Society for Paediatric Gastroenterology HaN, 2019; Krick et al., 1992; Rieken et al., 2011; Romano et al., 2017).

Protein needs in children with CP are generally similar to those of typically developing children, except in certain situations such as tube-fed, non-ambulant children. Protein intake may be inadequate when overall calorie intake is low, particularly in tube-fed children. In such cases, the DRI for protein in typically developing children can be used as a guideline to estimate requirements for children with CP. Supplementary protein may be indicated in specific clinical situations, including the presence of decubitus ulcers, low calorie intake, or severe undernutrition. For children with severe malnutrition, a protein intake of approximately 2.0 g/kg per day along with a 20% increase in total energy intake is typically sufficient to promote catch-up growth (Bell & Samson-Fang, 2013; European Society for Paediatric Gastroenterology HaN, 2019; Pencharz, 2010).

Requirements and Recommended Intake for Micronutrients

Micronutrient deficiencies are common in children with CP, particularly among those who are tube-fed. Deficiencies most often involve calcium, iron, zinc, vitamins C, D, and E, magnesium, selenium, copper, and manganese. Reduced energy intake, required to prevent overweight, frequently leads to insufficient micronutrient intake.

The ESPGHAN recommends applying the Dietary Reference Intakes (DRI) of typically developing children to guide micronutrient needs in this group. Iron supplementation is prioritized for children with deficiency, with RDAs of 10 mg/day (7–10 years), 12 mg/day (adolescent boys), and 15 mg/day (adolescent girls).

Special attention should be given to bone health, as impaired growth and increased fracture risk are common. Supplementation with calcium and vitamin D (800–1000 IU/day) is therefore essential. Adequate dietary fiber intake is also advised, following the formula: age plus 5 g/day for children older than 2 years. This point should be taken into account that identified deficiencies should be corrected either by incorporating nutrient-rich foods or, when necessary, through supplementation. Importantly, the treatment of confirmed deficiencies—verified by blood or serum analysis—often requires targeted supplementation beyond dietary measures (Campanozzi & Staiano, 2010; Carman et al., 2022; European Society for Paediatric Gastroenterology HaN, 2019; Prasad & Bhriguvanshi, 2022).

Fluids Requirements

Children with CP are at increased risk of dehydration due to factors such as impaired swallowing, drooling, inability to communicate thirst, and the use of hypercaloric formulas. Therefore, careful monitoring of hydration status is essential, with individualized assessment and adjustment of fluid intake to ensure adequate hydration. Fluid requirements are commonly estimated using actual body weight with the conventional Holliday-Segar equation; however, due to ongoing fluid losses through saliva, sweating, and respiratory evaporation, as well as limited oral intake, targeting approximately 90% of calculated fluid needs is often more practical and achievable in clinical practice (Azcue et al., 1996; European Society for Paediatric Gastroenterology HaN, 2019).

Enteral Tube Feeding

Enteral feeding is indicated for children with a functioning GI tract who cannot meet their nutritional needs by mouth, remain undernourished despite support, or struggle with significant swallowing and feeding problems. There are several ways to provide tube feeding, including nasogastric (NG), naso-jejunal, gastrostomy, gastrojejunostomy, and jejunostomy tubes (ABoDatCGT F., 2002; Dabydeen et al., 2008; Pentiuk et al., 2011; Vernon-Roberts et al., 2010; Nutrition: ECo et al., 2010).

The initial feed of choice for most children is a standard polymeric formula with an energy density of 1.0 kcal/mL. For those with higher energy requirements or poor tolerance to large feeding volumes, strategies such as using energy-dense formulas (1.5 kcal/mL) or adding glucose polymers and/or long-chain triglycerides can help increase caloric intake without overburdening the GI system. Conversely, in children with lower energy needs or rapid weight gain, a reduced-energy formula (0.75 kcal/mL) may be more appropriate to prevent overnutrition (Motil, 1994; Prasad & Bhriguvanshi, 2022).

Although enteral tube feeding is often essential for children with CP, it may be associated with certain complications. The most common issues include GI symptoms or inappropriate weight gain (Bell & Samson-Fang, 2013; Committee WFUE, 2007; Vernon-Roberts et al., 2010; Nutrition: ECo et al., 2010). A summary of potential complications and recommended management strategies is provided in the Box 5.3.

Box 5.3 Common Complications of Enteral Tube Feeding and Their Management

Constipation

- Ensure sufficient fluid and dietary fiber intake.
- Use fiber-enriched feeds or fiber supplements if needed.
- In some cases, laxative medication may still be required.

Vomiting and Regurgitation

- Confirm correct tube placement.
- Consider slower infusion rates, smaller frequent boluses, or upright positioning during feeds.
- If intolerance persists, post-pyloric feeding may be considered.
- Medical or surgical management for gastroesophageal reflux may be necessary.

Diarrhea

- Begin by reducing infusion rate or bolus size, or switch to continuous feeding.
- Use formulas with lower osmolarity and gradually increase as tolerated.
- In children with impaired gut function, a semi-elemental formula may be indicated.
- If due to contamination, ensure use of sterile commercial feeds, strict hygiene, and appropriate hang times.

Excessive Weight Gain

- Occurs when energy intake exceeds requirements.
- Strategies include reducing feed volume, switching to lower-energy density formulas (e.g., 0.75 kcal/mL), or using nutrient-dense formulas in smaller volumes.
- Protein and micronutrient supplementation may be needed in children with low energy intake, but care must be taken not to exceed safe upper limits.

5.4 Food and Drug Interaction

Several medications are involved in the management of CP to control symptoms and address associated complications. These may include drugs to reduce spasticity, involuntary movements, or seizures, as well as agents to improve comfort, posture, digestion, breathing, pain, and behavioral or learning difficulties.

Anticonvulsants may predispose patients to nutrient deficiencies such as vitamins D, B6, B12, K, folate, calcium, and biotin, while muscle relaxants (e.g., baclofen, dantrolene) can cause GI side effects including diarrhea, constipation, or weight changes. Benzodiazepines such as clonazepam may also induce drowsiness, dizziness, or GI complications. Supportive measures like appropriate laxative use, attention to fiber and fluid intake, and the use of probiotics can help manage constipation (Angelakou, n.d.; CerebralPalsy.org, n.d.; Mayo Clinic Staff, 2023; McCabe-Sellers et al., 2003). The most common medication that are used in CP along with their food–drug interaction illustrated in Table 5.1.

Table 5.1 Commonly prescribed medications for cerebral palsy and their food–drug interactions

Drug	Trade Name	Food–Drug Interactions
Anticholinergics		
Benztropine	Cogentin	**Side effects:** Loss of appetite and weight **Avoid:** Alcohol
Carbidopa/levodopa	Sinemet	**Side effects:** Hypokalemia, anorexia **Avoid:** Alcohol, high protein diets and avoid large fluctuations in daily protein, high-fiber diets, vitamin B6, and mineral supplements (Fe)
Glycopyrrolate	Robinul	**Avoid:** Alcohol
Procyclidine hydrochloride	Kemadrin	**Avoid:** Alcohol
Trihexyphenidyl hydrochloride	Artane	**Avoid:** Alcohol
Anticonvulsants		
Gabapentin	Neurontin	**Side effects:** Increase appetite and weight gain **Avoid:** Alcohol
Lamotrigine	Lamictal	**Side effects:** Decrease appetite, weight loss, and decreased availability of many nutrients **Avoid:** Alcohol
Oxcarbazepine	Trileptal	**Avoid:** Alcohol
Topiramate	Topamax	**Side effects:** Anorexia, weight loss, and decreased availability of many nutrients **Avoid:** Alcohol
Zonisamide	Zonegran	**Side effects:** Anorexia, weight loss, and decreased availability of many nutrients **Avoid:** Alcohol
Antidepressants		
Citalopram	Celexa	**Avoid:** St John's wort and alcohol
Escitalopram	Lexapro	**Avoid:** St John's wort and alcohol
Fluoxetine	Prozac	**Side effects:** Anorexia, hypokalemia **Avoid:** Alcohol
Paroxetine	Paxil	**Side effects:** Increase appetite **Avoid:** Alcohol, St John's wort
Sertraline	Zoloff	**Avoid:** Alcohol, St John's wort, and grapefruit or grapefruit juice
Antispastic		
Baclofen	Lioresal	**Avoid:** Alcohol
Diazepam	Valium	**Side effects:** Anorexia **Avoid:** Alcohol, grapefruit or grapefruit juice, and caffeine
Dantrolene	Dantrium	**Avoid:** Alcohol
Cyclobenzadrine	Flexeril	**Avoid:** Alcohol
Tizanidine	Zanaflex	**Avoid:** Alcohol, caffeine

Acknowledgments The authors confirm that the content, analysis, and conclusions of this manuscript are their own work. AI-based tools were used solely to assist in improving the clarity and correctness of the English language.

References

ABoDatCGT F. (2002). Guidelines for the use of parenteral and enteral nutrition in adult and pediatric patients. *JPEN Journal of Parenteral and Enteral Nutrition, 26*, 1SA–138SA.

Alenazi, K. A. (2022). Vitamin D deficiency in children with cerebral palsy: A narrative review of epidemiology, contributing factors, clinical consequences and interventions. *Saudi Journal of Biological Sciences, 29*(4), 2007–2013.

Angelakou, I. A. (n.d.). *Food-drug interactions and their impact on the pharmacotherapy.*

Azcue, M. P., Zello, G. A., Levy, L. D., & Pencharz, P. B. (1996). Energy expenditure and body composition in children with spastic quadriplegic cerebral palsy. *The Journal of Pediatrics, 129*(6), 870–876.

Barkoudah, E., & Glader, L. (2019). *Cerebral palsy: Epidemiology, etiology, and prevention.* Recuperado de. https://www.uptodate.com/home

Bell, K., & Samson-Fang, L. (2013). Nutritional management of children with cerebral palsy. *European Journal of Clinical Nutrition, 67*(2), S13–SS6.

Benfer, K. A., Weir, K. A., Bell, K. L., Ware, R. S., Davies, P. S., & Boyd, R. N. (2017). Oropharyngeal dysphagia and cerebral palsy. *Pediatrics, 140*(6), e20170731.

Campanozzi, A., & Staiano, A. (2010). Impact of malnutrition on gastrointestinal disorders and gross motor abilities in children with cerebral palsy. *Brain and Development, 32*(2), 168.

Carman, K. B., Aydın, K., Kilic Aydin, B., Cansu, A., Direk, M. C., Durmus, S., et al. (2022). Evaluation of micronutrient levels in children with cerebral palsy. *Pediatrics International, 64*(1), e15005.

Center BI. (2023). *Cerebral palsy & nutrition.* https://birthinjurycenter.org/cerebral-palsy/nutrition

Cerebral Palsy Alliance Research Foundation. (n.d.). *Gross motor function classification system (GMFCS).* https://cparf.org/what-is-cerebral-palsy/severity-of-cerebral-palsy/gross-motor-function-classification-system-gmfcs

CerebralPalsy.org. (n.d.). *Medication and drug therapy.* https://www.cerebralpalsy.org/about-cerebral-palsy/treatment/medication

Cleveland Clinic. (2025). *Cerebral palsy.* Retrieved August 16, 2023, from https://my.clevelandclinic.org/health/diseases/8717-cerebral-palsy

Committee WFUE. (2007). *Protein and amino acid requirements in human nutrition.*

Culley, W. J., & Middleton TO. (1969). Caloric requirements of mentally retarded children with and without motor dysfunction. *The Journal of Pediatrics, 75*(3), 380–384.

Dabydeen, L., Thomas, J. E., Aston, T. J., Hartley, H., Sinha, S. K., & Eyre, J. A. (2008). High-energy and-protein diet increases brain and corticospinal tract growth in term and preterm infants after perinatal brain injury. *Pediatrics, 121*(1), 148–156.

Del Giudice, E., Staiano, A., Capano, G., Romano, A., Florimonte, L., Miele, E., et al. (1999). Gastrointestinal manifestations in children with cerebral palsy. *Brain and Development, 21*(5), 307–311.

Edvinsson, S. E., & Lundqvist, L. O. (2016). Prevalence of orofacial dysfunction in cerebral palsy and its association with gross motor function and manual ability. *Developmental Medicine and Child Neurology, 58*(4), 385–394.

Erkin, G., Culha, C., Ozel, S., & Kirbiyik, E. G. (2010). Feeding and gastrointestinal problems in children with cerebral palsy. *International Journal of Rehabilitation Research, 33*(3), 218–224.

Erlichman, M. (1989). The role of speech language pathologists in the management of dysphagia, 1989. *Health Technology Assessment Reports, 1*, 1–10.

European Society for Paediatric Gastroenterology HaN. (2019). *Recommendations for nutritional management of children with neurological impairment (NI)*. ESPGHAN.

Fahey, M. C., Maclennan, A. H., Kretzschmar, D., Gecz, J., & Kruer, M. C. (2017). The genetic basis of cerebral palsy. *Developmental Medicine and Child Neurology, 59*(5), 462–469.

Graham, D., Paget, S. P., & Wimalasundera, N. (2019). Current thinking in the health care management of children with cerebral palsy. *Medical Journal of Australia, 210*(3), 129–135.

Houlihan, C. M. (2014). Bone health in cerebral palsy: Who's at risk and what to do about it? *Journal of Pediatric Rehabilitation Medicine, 7*(2), 143–153.

Jahan, I., Muhit, M., Hardianto, D., Laryea, F., Chhetri, A. B., Smithers-Sheedy, H., et al. (2021). Epidemiology of cerebral palsy in low-and middle-income countries: Preliminary findings from an international multi-centre cerebral palsy register. *Developmental Medicine and Child Neurology, 63*(11), 1327–1336.

Jesus, A. O., & Stevenson, R. D. (2020). Optimizing nutrition and bone health in children with cerebral palsy. *Physical Medicine and Rehabilitation Clinics, 31*(1), 25–37.

Junges, C., Machado, T. D., Nunes Filho, P. R. S., Riesgo, R., & Mello, E. D. (2020). Deficiência de vitamina D em pacientes pediátricos que fazem uso de fármacos antiepilépticos-revisão sistemática com metanálise. *Jornal de Pediatria, 96*, 559–568.

Kim, J.-S., Han, Z.-A., Song, D. H., Oh, H.-M., & Chung, M. E. (2013). Characteristics of dysphagia in children with cerebral palsy, related to gross motor function. *American Journal of Physical Medicine & Rehabilitation, 92*(10), 912–919.

Korzeniewski, S. J., Slaughter, J., Lenski, M., Haak, P., & Paneth, N. (2018). The complex aetiology of cerebral palsy. *Nature Reviews Neurology, 14*(9), 528–543.

Krick, J., Murphy, P. E., Markham, J. F., & Shapiro, B. K. (1992). A proposed formula for calculating energy needs of children with cerebral palsy. *Developmental Medicine and Child Neurology, 34*(6), 481–487.

Kuperminc, M. N., & Stevenson, R. D. (2008). Growth and nutrition disorders in children with cerebral palsy. *Developmental Disabilities Research Reviews, 14*(2), 137–146.

Le Roy, C., Barja, S., Sepúlveda, C., Guzmán, M., Olivarez, M., Figueroa, M., et al. (2021). Deficiencia de vitamina D y de hierro en niños y adolescentes con parálisis cerebral. *Neurología, 36*(2), 112–118.

MacLennan, A. H., Thompson, S. C., & Gecz, J. (2015). Cerebral palsy: Causes, pathways, and the role of genetic variants. *American Journal of Obstetrics and Gynecology, 213*(6), 779–788.

Mayo Clinic Staff. (2023). *Cerebral palsy—Diagnosis and treatment.* https://www.mayoclinic.org/diseases-conditions/cerebral-palsy/diagnosis-treatment/drc-20354005

McCabe-Sellers, B., Frankel, E. H., & Wolfe, J. J. (2003). *Handbook of food-drug interactions*. CRC Press.

McIntyre, S., Goldsmith, S., Webb, A., Ehlinger, V., Hollung, S. J., McConnell, K., et al. (2022). Global prevalence of cerebral palsy: A systematic analysis. *Developmental Medicine and Child Neurology, 64*(12), 1494–1506.

McMichael, G., Bainbridge, M., Haan, E., Corbett, M., Gardner, A., Thompson, S., et al. (2015). Whole-exome sequencing points to considerable genetic heterogeneity of cerebral palsy. *Molecular Psychiatry, 20*(2), 176–182.

Modlesky, C. M., & Zhang, C. (2020). Complicated muscle-bone interactions in children with cerebral palsy. *Current Osteoporosis Reports, 18*(1), 47–56.

Moreno-De-Luca, A., Ledbetter, D. H., & Martin, C. L. (2012). Genetic insights into the causes and classification of the cerebral palsies. *The Lancet Neurology, 11*(3), 283–292.

Moreno-De-Luca, A., Millan, F., Pesacreta, D. R., Elloumi, H. Z., Oetjens, M. T., Teigen, C., et al. (2021). Molecular diagnostic yield of exome sequencing in patients with cerebral palsy. *JAMA, 325*(5), 467–475.

Motil, K. J. (1994). Enteral nutrition in the neurologically impaired child. In *Pediatric enteral nutrition* (pp. 217–237). Chapman & Hall.

Mus-Peters, C. T., Huisstede, B. M., Noten, S., Hitters, M. W., van der Slot, W. M., & van den Berg-Emons, R. J. (2019). Low bone mineral density in ambulatory persons with cerebral palsy? A systematic review. *Disability and Rehabilitation, 41*(20), 2392–2402.

NHS. (2023). *Cerebral palsy—Symptoms*. Retrieved May 31, 2023, from https://www.nhs.uk/conditions/cerebral-palsy/symptoms

NINDS. (2025). *Cerebral palsy*. Retrieved March 20, 2025, from https://www.ninds.nih.gov/health-information/disorders/cerebral-palsy

Nutrition: ECo, Braegger, C., Decsi, T., Dias, J. A., Hartman, C., Kolaček, S., et al. (2010). Practical approach to paediatric enteral nutrition: A comment by the ESPGHAN committee on nutrition. *Journal of Pediatric Gastroenterology and Nutrition, 51*(1), 110–122.

Oskoui, M., Coutinho, F., Dykeman, J., Jetté, N., & Pringsheim, T. (2013). An update on the prevalence of cerebral palsy: A systematic review and meta-analysis. *Developmental Medicine and Child Neurology, 55*(6), 509–519.

Pencharz, P. (2010). Protein and energy requirements for 'optimal'catch-up growth. *European Journal of Clinical Nutrition, 64*(1), S5–S7.

Pentiuk, S., O'Flaherty, T., Santoro, K., Willging, P., & Kaul, A. (2011). Pureed by gastrostomy tube diet improves gagging and retching in children with fundoplication. *Journal of Parenteral and Enteral Nutrition, 35*(3), 375–379.

Potcovaru, C. G., Salmen, T., Chitu, M. C., Dima, V., Mihai, M. B., Bohiltea, R. E., et al. (2022). Cerebral palsy: Review of epidemiology, etiology, clinical features, classification and prevention. *Romanian Journal of Pediatrics, 71*(S2), 18–22.

Prasad, D., & Bhriguvanshi, A. (2022). Nutritional issues and management in children with cerebral palsy. *Ann Pediatr Child Health., 10*(3), 1271.

Rieken, R., van Goudoever, J. B., Schierbeek, H., Willemsen, S. P., Calis, E. A., Tibboel, D., et al. (2011). Measuring body composition and energy expenditure in children with severe neurologic impairment and intellectual disability. *The American Journal of Clinical Nutrition, 94*(3), 759–766.

Romano, C., van Wynckel, M., Hulst, J., Broekaert, I., Bronsky, J., Dall'Oglio, L., et al. (2017). European society for paediatric gastroenterology, hepatology and nutrition guidelines for the evaluation and treatment of gastrointestinal and nutritional complications in children with neurological impairment. *Journal of Pediatric Gastroenterology and Nutrition, 65*(2), 242–264.

Rosenbaum, P., Paneth, N., Leviton, A., Goldstein, M., Bax, M., Damiano, D., et al. (2007). A report: The definition and classification of cerebral palsy April 2006. *Developmental Medicine and Child Neurology. Supplement, 109*(suppl 109), 8–14.

Rouabhi, A., Husein, N., Dewey, D., Letourneau, N., Daboval, T., Oskoui, M., et al. (2023). Development of a bedside tool to predict the diagnosis of cerebral palsy in term-born neonates. *JAMA Pediatrics, 177*(2), 177–186.

Rouster, A. S., Karpinski, A. C., Silver, D., Monagas, J., & Hyman, P. E. (2016). Functional gastrointestinal disorders dominate pediatric gastroenterology outpatient practice. *Journal of Pediatric Gastroenterology and Nutrition, 62*(6), 847–851.

Schaefer, G. B. (Ed.). (2008). Genetics considerations in cerebral palsy. *Seminars in Pediatric Neurology, 15*, 21. Elsevier.

Trivić, I., & Hojsak, I. (2019). Evaluation and treatment of malnutrition and associated gastrointestinal complications in children with cerebral palsy. *Pediatric Gastroenterology, Hepatology & Nutrition, 22*(2), 122–131.

Van Naarden, B. K., Doernberg, N., Schieve, L., Christensen, D., Goodman, A., & Yeargin-Allsopp, M. (2016). Birth prevalence of cerebral palsy: A population-based study. *Pediatrics, 137*(1), e20152872.

Vernon-Roberts, A., Wells, J., Grant, H., Alder, N., Vadamalayan, B., Eltumi, M., et al. (2010). Gastrostomy feeding in cerebral palsy: Enough and no more. *Developmental Medicine and Child Neurology, 52*(12), 1099–1105.

Yi, Y. G., Oh, B.-M., Seo, H. G., Shin, H.-I., & Bang, M. S. (2019). Dysphagia-related quality of life in adults with cerebral palsy on full oral diet without enteral nutrition. *Dysphagia, 34*(2), 201–209.

Chapter 6
Attention-Deficit/Hyperactivity Disorder

Abstract

- Attention-Deficit/Hyperactivity Disorder (ADHD) is a disabling neurodevelopmental disorder affecting about 8% of children worldwide, presenting as inattentive, hyperactive-impulsive, or combined type, and often associated with significant psychiatric comorbidities and functional impairment.
- ADHD results from complex interactions of genetic predisposition, prenatal and perinatal insults, nutritional deficiencies, and environmental toxin exposures that disrupt neurodevelopment.
- Stimulant medications commonly used for ADHD may suppress appetite, leading to reduced caloric intake, inadequate growth, and potential impact on final height and bone health.
- Nutritional management emphasizes balanced, nutrient-dense diets rich in fruits, vegetables, whole grains, lean protein, and healthy fats, with regular meals and snacks while limiting processed and sugar-rich foods.
- Mediterranean and DASH dietary patterns are associated with reduced symptom severity, whereas elimination diets (REDs, Feingold) may benefit selected children but require professional supervision to avoid nutritional deficiencies.
- Supplementation with omega-3 fatty acids, iron, zinc, vitamin D, magnesium, folate, and vitamin B12 may improve behavioral and cognitive outcomes in deficient children.
- Children with ADHD often exhibit altered trace element profiles, including low zinc, ferritin, magnesium, and an increased copper-to-zinc ratio.
- It is recommended to minimize exposure to lead, pesticides, and PCBs, ensure safe food handling practices, and encourage regular physical activity to support optimal neurodevelopment and reduce ADHD risk.
- Food–drug interactions are clinically important; ADHD medications (stimulants, non-stimulants, antidepressants) may interact with caffeine, alcohol, or grapefruit juice, requiring careful monitoring for safety and effectiveness.

M. H. Rouhani et al., *The Healing Plate*, SpringerBriefs in Modern Perspectives on Disability Research, https://doi.org/10.1007/978-981-95-8150-4_6

Keywords Attention-deficit/hyperactivity disorder (ADHD) · Neurodevelopmental disorders · Nutrition · Dietary patterns · Micronutrients · Stimulant medications · Growth and bone health · Trace elements · Environmental toxins · Food–drug interactions

6.1 Definition and Epidemiology

Attention-Deficit/Hyperactivity Disorder (ADHD) is a neurodevelopmental disability disorder characterized by core deficits in attention and behavior, typically emerging in childhood and often persisting into adulthood (Sharma & Couture, 2014). Clinically, ADHD manifests in three forms, predominantly inattentive, predominantly hyperactive-impulsive, and combined type, according to the DSM-5 (American Psychiatric Association, 1994). The disorder profoundly impairs daily functioning, increases susceptibility to psychiatric comorbidities, and imposes substantial societal and economic burdens, highlighting its disabling nature and the imperative for early, comprehensive, and integrative management (Asherson et al., 2012; Gupte-Singh et al., 2017; Katzman et al., 2017; Zhao et al., 2019; Zulauf et al., 2014).

Globally, ADHD affects approximately 8% of children and adolescents (Ayano et al., 2023). In the United States, an estimated 7 million children (11.4%) aged 3–17 years have been diagnosed with ADHD at some point in their lives (Danielson et al., 2022). The inattentive subtype (ADHD-I) is the most common, followed by hyperactive (ADHD-HI) and combined (ADHD-C) types (Ayano et al., 2023). Boys are nearly twice as likely as girls to receive a diagnosis, and prevalence varies across racial and ethnic groups, being highest among Black, White, and American Indian/ Alaska Native children. Overall, non-Hispanic children are diagnosed more frequently than Hispanic children (Danielson et al., 2024). Notably, nearly two-thirds of affected children present with at least one comorbid behavioral or psychiatric disorder (Mahone & Denckla, 2017).

6.2 Etiology

ADHD is a multifactorial neurodevelopmental disability disorder arising from the interplay of genetic, prenatal, nutritional, and environmental factors. Genetic heritability accounts for nearly three-quarters of the risk, with polygenic variants in dopaminergic and serotonergic pathways (e.g., *DRD4*, *DAT1*, *SNAP25*, *SLC6A3*) identified through twin studies and GWAS (Poddar et al., 2025). However, genetics alone are insufficient; prenatal and perinatal insults, including maternal stress, malnutrition, inflammation, preterm birth, preeclampsia, and birth asphyxia, further disrupt neurodevelopment (Getahun et al., 2013; Vohr et al., 2017). Nutritional deficiencies such as iron, vitamin D, and omega-3 fatty acids impair functional ability, neurotransmission, and brain connectivity (Khoshbakht et al., 2018; Verlaet et al., 2014). Additionally, maternal substance use, environmental toxins, and early life exposures amplify susceptibility (Maher et al., 2024). Thus, ADHD reflects the dynamic interaction of genetic predisposition with environmental and nutritional influences, explaining its heterogeneity and guiding preventive and therapeutic strategies (Cortese & Coghill, 2018; Nilsen & Tulve, 2020; Wermter et al., 2010).

6.3 Nutritional Managements

6.3.1 Nutritional Challenges

The central nutritional goal in ADHD children is to provide adequate energy intake to support normal growth and active participation in therapeutic programs. Stimulant medications, which are widely prescribed in this population, frequently induce appetite suppression. This effect may result in reduced caloric consumption, inadequate weight gain, and compromised linear growth (Richardson et al., 2017). With long-term use, such treatments have additionally been associated with reduced final adult height and potential adverse consequences for bone mineralization (Richardson et al., 2017).

6.3.2 General Dietary Recommendations

Nutritional management of ADHD emphasizes the importance of overall dietary patterns and lifestyle behaviors rather than isolated nutrient intake (Lange, 2020; Lange et al., 2022). The relationship between diet and ADHD is complex and often reciprocal; evidence from prospective studies indicates that ADHD symptoms may shape subsequent dietary quality more strongly than diet determines symptom severity (Mian et al., 2019). For instance, higher sugar intake observed in some children is suggested by longitudinal data to represent a behavioral consequence of ADHD rather than a causal factor (Del-Ponte et al., 2019). Despite these uncertainties, maintaining a balanced, nutrient-dense diet is essential, as optimal diet quality may support both behavioral regulation and cognitive ability. Importantly, children with ADHD often exhibit lower adherence to healthy dietary patterns, characterized by high consumption of fruits, vegetables, whole grains, and lean proteins, and greater intake of sugar-rich, processed, and Western-style foods (Lee et al., 2022; Rojo-Marticella et al., 2022; Ryu et al., 2022), while frequently showing inadequate intake of protein, vitamins B1, B2, C, calcium, and zinc (Salvat et al., 2022). Overall, dietary recommendations should integrate an evaluation of the child's nutritional status, eating behaviors, and the potential influence of pharmacological treatments on appetite and food intake.

6.3.3 Recommended Dietary Patterns

Healthy Dietary Patterns: Diet quality strongly modulates ADHD risk and symptom severity in children. Diets high in refined sugars, saturated fats, and ultra-processed foods such as Western-style and "junk food" diets exacerbate hyperactivity and inattention, whereas nutrient-dense patterns, rich in vegetables, fruits, legumes, whole grains, fish, nuts, and low-fat dairy, are protective. Nutrients such as omega-3 fatty acids, polyunsaturated fats, iron, zinc, magnesium, and phytochemicals support cognitive function, attention, and behavioral regulation. Adherence to Mediterranean or DASH dietary patterns consistently correlates with improved behavioral outcomes, reduced symptom severity, and lower ADHD prevalence. A balanced diet providing sufficient carbohydrates for brain energy, high-quality proteins, and consistent micronutrient intake remains a cornerstone of dietary management in ADHD (Darabi et al., 2022; Del-Ponte et al., 2019; Khoshbakht et al., 2021; Lee et al., 2022; San Mauro Martin et al., 2021).

Elimination Diets: Restricted elimination diets (REDs) and oligoantigenic diets can improve symptoms in some ADHD children, though they carry risks of nutritional deficiencies and are challenging to maintain (Pelsser et al., 2009). These diets involve eliminating potential dietary triggers (e.g., eggs, nuts, wheat, dairy, soy/tofu, chocolate, dyes, corn) and foods with artificial additives, followed by systematic reintroduction to identify triggers. The elimination phase typically lasts 2–3 weeks, with daily behavioral monitoring. Foods suspected of causing symptoms, such as artificial colorings, preservatives, corn, soy, citrus, and commonly consumed beverages, are avoided, while fresh meat, poultry, most vegetables, non-citrus fruits, rice, and oats are allowed. Reintroduction is done one item at a time over several days, with careful observation for behavioral or allergic responses. Elimination diets are particularly promising in younger children and those with comorbid allergic or atopic conditions Optimal outcomes require dietitian supervision to ensure nutritional adequacy, allergist assessment for children with atopic tendencies, and targeted daily micronutrient supplementation to prevent deficiencies (Jacobson & Schardt, 1999).

Feingold diet: The Feingold diet, which eliminates artificial colors, flavors, and salicylates, may reduce hyperactivity in sensitive individuals, although the overall evidence is inconsistent (Feingold, 1975; Kavale & Forness, 1983; Nigg et al., 2012; Schab & Trinh, 2004). Modern adaptations primarily focus on removing artificial additives and dyes, and dietary adjustments should be individualized for children who demonstrate sensitivity (see Fig. 6.1 for lists of avoided and allowed foods according to Feingold diet).

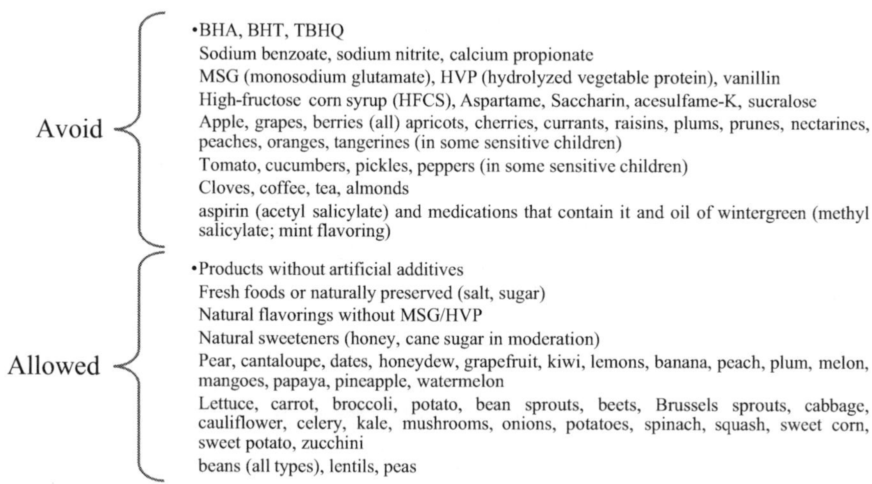

Fig. 6.1 Lists of avoided and allowed foods according to Feingold diet.

6.3.4 Targeted Nutrients and Supplements

Omega-3 Fatty Acids: Children with ADHD often have low serum long-chain polyunsaturated fatty acids, which may contribute to hyperactivity (Chang et al., 2016; Chang et al., 2018; Ramakrishnan et al., 2016). Omega-3 fatty acids are generally safe, though minor gastrointestinal effects and interactions with anticoagulants or NSAIDs can occur.

Iron and Zinc: Iron and zinc deficiencies are linked to greater ADHD severity, cognitive deficits, and poorer treatment response; Meanwhile, supplementation in deficient children can enhance behavioral and cognitive outcomes (Abdullah et al., 2019; Chen et al., 2013; Granero et al., 2021; Lozoff et al., 2014).

Vitamin D and Magnesium: Children with ADHD frequently present with lower serum 25-hydroxyvitamin D levels. Supplementation may modestly improve hyperactivity, inattention, and overall behavior, especially when combined with methylphenidate (Gan et al., 2019; Kotsi et al., 2019). Lower magnesium levels are also observed in ADHD, and combined supplementation of vitamin D and magnesium has shown enhanced outcomes (Hemamy et al., 2021).

Folate and Vitamin B12: Deficiency of vitamin B12 or folate, particularly in individuals with MTHFR mutations or elevated homocysteine, may worsen psychiatric symptoms, including ADHD. Correcting these deficiencies is essential for optimizing clinical outcomes and supporting effective management (Bhatia & Singh, 2015).

Probiotics: Emerging evidence suggests potential benefit of probiotic supplementation, particularly with Lactobacillus rhamnosus, though findings remain inconsistent (Kumperscak et al., 2020).

6.3.5 *Trace Element Alterations*

Studies on children with ADHD indicate notable alterations in trace elements. Blood analyses consistently show reduced levels of zinc, ferritin, and magnesium, and chromium, alongside an increased copper-to-zinc ratio compared to controls. Meanwhile evidence on copper remains inconsistent across biological samples. (Mahmoud et al., 2011; Skalny et al., 2020). In contrast, hair mineral analyses reveal significant reductions in magnesium and manganese, with lower hair zinc and magnesium inversely associated with symptom severity (Skalny et al., 2020).

6.3.6 *Practical Supplementation Considerations*

As with all children, supplementation with vitamins such as A and C may be necessary in cases of restricted dietary variety or elevated risk of deficiency. Universal recommendations include daily supplementation of 10 mcg (400 IU) vitamin D for all children, particularly during autumn and winter months. A practical approach favors the use of age-appropriate over-the-counter multivitamins rather than high-dose individual supplements (East & North Hertfordshire NHS Trust, n.d.).

6.3.7 *Other Considerations*

- **Food Safety and Environmental Toxins in ADHD:** Exposure to environmental toxins, including lead, pesticide residues, polychlorinated biphenyls (PCBs), and manganese, has been linked to ADHD pathogenesis. Early life exposure to organophosphate and organochlorine pesticides is strongly associated with impaired neurodevelopment and increased ADHD risk, with prenatal and infant exposures being particularly harmful (Bouchard et al., 2010; Hertz-Picciotto et al., 2018). PCBs contribute to ADHD-related behavioral disturbances, higher body mass index, and reduced IQ, while manganese toxicity is associated with increased incidence of attention deficit disorder and adverse infant outcomes (Lopez-Garcia et al., 2025; O'Neal & Zheng, 2015). Minimizing exposure to these toxins is therefore critical for supporting optimal neurodevelopment and reducing ADHD risk.
- **Sugar and sweeteners:** No strong evidence supports a causal link between sugar or aspartame and ADHD symptoms (Heilskov Rytter et al., 2015; Millichap & Yee, 2012), although parents often report worsening hyperactivity following consumption of high sugar or aspartame loads. Higher sugar intake observed in some children is suggested by longitudinal data to represent a behavioral consequence of ADHD rather than a causal factor.

- **Maternal diet:** Higher maternal diet quality during pregnancy is associated with modest reductions in ADHD risk in offspring (Katzman et al., 2017). Optimal maternal nutrition during gestation is associated with lower ADHD symptom scores and a reduced likelihood of diagnosis by 8 years of age. By contrast, the quality of diet during early childhood appears to have a less pronounced impact on subsequent ADHD outcomes (Borge et al., 2021).
- **Ketogenic Diet:** While beneficial in epilepsy, the ketogenic diet has shown no specific advantage for ADHD and is not recommended (Bostock et al., 2017). It is noteworthy that children with epilepsy frequently exhibit ADHD, and children with ADHD often display electroencephalographic changes.

6.3.8 Recommendations

- Encourage regular meal patterns with small, frequent healthy snacks, emphasizing breakfast and bedtime meals.
- Offer preferred foods alongside one or two new items to expand taste preferences.
- Monitor medication-related appetite suppression and adjust meals/snacks accordingly.
- Include starchy carbohydrates at each meal (potatoes, bread, rice, pasta, cereals), preferably wholegrain or high-fiber varieties.
- Ensure adequate protein intake at lunch and dinner, from diverse sources including beans, pulses, fish, eggs, meat, and poultry.
- Include dairy products for calcium to support bone and dental health.
- Use unsaturated oils and spreads (e.g., vegetable, rapeseed, olive oils) in moderation.
- Maintain adequate hydration, limiting fruit juices and sugar-sweetened beverages.
- Consider supplementation with omega-3, iron, zinc, vitamin D, and magnesium when deficiencies are identified or dietary variety is limited.
- Implement elimination diets cautiously, targeting artificial colorings and additives, under close nutritional and clinical supervision.
- Educate families on balanced eating, food safety (e.g., lead exposure, proper food handling), and reducing mealtime distractions.
- Avoid unproven megavitamin or restrictive regimens that may compromise nutrition.
- Specific food safety measures: flush cold tap water for 2 min if lead contamination is suspected; discard foods left at room temperature > 2 h or > 1 h if the temperature is over 90 ° F.
- Encourage routine moderate-to-vigorous physical activity, which improves cognitive, behavioral, and physical symptoms (Ng et al., 2017).
- Ensure appropriate weight gain and growth, particularly when appetite is reduced; snacks can support this goal.

6.4 Food and Drug Interaction

ADHD medications are used to manage symptoms such as hyperactivity, impulsivity, and reduced attention span. These drugs, which include stimulants, non-stimulants, and sometimes antidepressants, work by increasing brain neurotransmitters like dopamine and norepinephrine. Finding the right medication and dose can take time, as individuals may respond differently and experience side effects that require adjustment. It is important to inform healthcare providers about all prescription drugs, over-the-counter medications, supplements, and caffeine intake, as combining substances may affect medication safety and effectiveness (Angelakou, n.d.; Cleveland Clinic, 2022). The most common medication that are used in ADHD along with their food–drug interaction is illustrated in Table 6.1.

Table 6.1 Commonly Prescribed Medications for Attention-deficit Hyperactivity Disorder and Their Food–Drug Interactions

Drug	Trade Name	Food–Drug Interactions
Stimulants		
Dexmethylphenidate	Focalin	**Side effects:** Anorexia **Avoid:** Limit caffeine intake
Methylphenidate	Ritalin	**Side effects:** Anorexia and weight loss, **Avoid:** Caffeine, alcohol
Dextroamphetamine mixed salts and amphetamine	Adderall	**Side effects:** Anorexia **Avoid:** Caffeine, alcohol
Methamphetamine	Desoxyn	**Side effects:** Anorexia **Avoid:** Caffeine, alcohol
Amphetamine	Evekeo	**Side effects:** Anorexia **Avoid:** Caffeine, alcohol
Dextroamphetamine	Zenzedi	**Side effects:** Anorexia **Avoid:** Caffeine, alcohol
Lisdexamfetamine dimesylate	Vyvanse	**Side effects:** Anorexia **Avoid:** Caffeine, alcohol
Non-stimulants		
Atomoxetine	Strattera	**Side effects:** Anorexia **Avoid:** Caffeine, alcohol
Viloxazine	Qelbree	**Side effects:** Anorexia **Avoid:** Caffeine, alcohol
Clonidine	Kapvay	**Side effects:**– **Avoid:** Alcohol
Guanfacine	Intuniv	**Side effects:** Anorexia **Avoid:** Grapefruit or grapefruit juice, alcohol

(continued)

Table 6.1 (continued)

Drug	Trade Name	Food–Drug Interactions
Antidepressant		
Bupropion	Wellbutrin	**Side effects:** Anorexia and weight loss **Avoid:** Alcohol
Desipramine	Norpramin	**Side effects:** Increased appetite **Avoid:** Alcohol
Imipramine	Tofranil	**Side effects:** Increased appetite **Avoid:** Alcohol
Nortriptyline	Pamelor	**Side effects:**– **Avoid:** Alcohol

Acknowledgments The authors confirm that the content, analysis, and conclusions of this manuscript are their own work. AI-based tools were used solely to assist in improving the clarity and correctness of the English language.

References

Abdullah, M., Jowett, B., Whittaker, P. J., & Patterson, L. (2019). The effectiveness of omega-3 supplementation in reducing ADHD associated symptoms in children as measured by the Conners' rating scales: A systematic review of randomized controlled trials. *Journal of Psychiatric Research, 110*, 64–73.

American Psychiatric Association (Ed.). (1994). *DSM-IV: Diagnostic and statistical manual of mental disorders* (4th ed.). American Psychiatric Association.

Angelakou, I. A. (n.d.). *Food-drug interactions and their impact on the pharmacotherapy.*

Asherson, P., Akehurst, R., Kooij, J. J., Huss, M., Beusterien, K., Sasané, R., et al. (2012). Under diagnosis of adult ADHD: Cultural influences and societal burden. *Journal of Attention Disorders, 16*(5 Suppl), 20s–38s.

Ayano, G., Demelash, S., Gizachew, Y., Tsegay, L., & Alati, R. (2023). The global prevalence of attention deficit hyperactivity disorder in children and adolescents: An umbrella review of meta-analyses. *Journal of Affective Disorders, 339*, 860–866.

Bhatia, P., & Singh, N. (2015). Homocysteine excess: Delineating the possible mechanism of neurotoxicity and depression. *Fundamental & Clinical Pharmacology, 29*(6), 522–528.

Borge, T. C., Biele, G., Papadopoulou, E., Andersen, L. F., Jacka, F., Eggesbø, M., et al. (2021). The associations between maternal and child diet quality and child ADHD—Findings from a large Norwegian pregnancy cohort study. *BMC Psychiatry, 21*(1), 139.

Bostock, E. C., Kirkby, K. C., & Taylor, B. V. (2017). The current status of the ketogenic diet in psychiatry. *Frontiers in Psychiatry, 8*, 43.

Bouchard, M. F., Bellinger, D. C., Wright, R. O., & Weisskopf, M. G. (2010). Attention-deficit/hyperactivity disorder and urinary metabolites of organophosphate pesticides. *Pediatrics, 125*(6), e1270–e1277.

Chang, J., Jingling, L., Huang, Y.-T., Lu, Y.-J., & Su, K.-P. (2016). Delay aversion, temporal processing, and N-3 fatty acids intake in children with attention-deficit/hyperactivity disorder (ADHD). *Clinical Psychological Science, 4*, 1094.

Chang, J. P., Su, K. P., Mondelli, V., & Pariante, C. M. (2018). Omega-3 polyunsaturated fatty acids in youths with attention deficit hyperactivity disorder: A systematic review and meta-analysis of clinical trials and biological studies. *Neuropsychopharmacology, 43*(3), 534–545.

Chen, M. H., Su, T. P., Chen, Y. S., Hsu, J. W., Huang, K. L., Chang, W. H., et al. (2013). Association between psychiatric disorders and iron deficiency anemia among children and adolescents: A nationwide population-based study. *BMC Psychiatry, 13*, 161.

Cleveland Clinic. (2022). *ADHD medication: How they work & side effects*. Cleveland Clinic. Retrieved June 10, 2022, from https://my.clevelandclinic.org/health/treatments/11766-adhd-medication

Cortese, S., & Coghill, D. (2018). Twenty years of research on attention-deficit/hyperactivity disorder (ADHD): Looking back, looking forward. *Evidence-Based Mental Health, 21*(4), 173–176.

Danielson, M. L., Claussen, A. H., Bitsko, R. H., Katz, S. M., Newsome, K., Blumberg, S. J., et al. (2024). ADHD prevalence among U.S. children and adolescents in 2022: Diagnosis, severity, co-occurring disorders, and treatment. *Journal of Clinical Child and Adolescent Psychology, 53*(3), 343–360.

Danielson, M. L., Holbrook, J. R., Bitsko, R. H., Newsome, K., Charania, S. N., McCord, R. F., et al. (2022). State-level estimates of the prevalence of parent-reported ADHD diagnosis and treatment among U.S. children and adolescents, 2016 to 2019. *Journal of Attention Disorders, 26*(13), 1685–1697.

Darabi, Z., Vasmehjani, A. A., Darand, M., Sangouni, A. A., & Hosseinzadeh, M. (2022). Adherence to Mediterranean diet and attention-deficit/hyperactivity disorder in children: A case control study. *Clin Nutr ESPEN, 47*, 346–350.

Del-Ponte, B., Anselmi, L., Assunção, M. C. F., Tovo-Rodrigues, L., Munhoz, T. N., Matijasevich, A., et al. (2019). Sugar consumption and attention-deficit/hyperactivity disorder (ADHD): A birth cohort study. *Journal of Affective Disorders, 243*, 290–296.

Del-Ponte, B., Quinte, G. C., Cruz, S., Grellert, M., & Santos, I. S. (2019). Dietary patterns and attention deficit/hyperactivity disorder (ADHD): A systematic review and meta-analysis. *Journal of Affective Disorders, 252*, 160–173.

East & North Hertfordshire NHS Trust. (n.d.). *Eating well with ADHD: East & North Hertfordshire NHS trust*. https://www.enherts-tr.nhs.uk/wp-content/uploads/2019/12/ADHD-leaflet-first-line-advice-updated-1-PDF-2.pdf

Feingold, B. F. (1975). Hyperkinesis and learning disabilities linked to artificial food flavors and colors. *The American Journal of Nursing, 75*(5), 797–803.

Gan, J., Galer, P., Ma, D., Chen, C., & Xiong, T. (2019). The effect of vitamin d supplementation on attention-deficit/hyperactivity disorder: A systematic review and meta-analysis of randomized controlled trials. *Journal of Child and Adolescent Psychopharmacology, 29*(9), 670–687.

Getahun, D., Rhoads, G. G., Demissie, K., Lu, S. E., Quinn, V. P., Fassett, M. J., et al. (2013). In utero exposure to ischemic-hypoxic conditions and attention-deficit/hyperactivity disorder. *Pediatrics, 131*(1), e53–e61.

Granero, R., Pardo-Garrido, A., Carpio-Toro, I. L., Ramírez-Coronel, A. A., Martínez-Suárez, P. C., & Reivan-Ortiz, G. G. (2021). The role of iron and zinc in the treatment of ADHD among children and adolescents: A systematic review of randomized clinical trials. *Nutrients, 13*(11), 4059.

Gupte-Singh, K., Singh, R. R., & Lawson, K. A. (2017). Economic burden of attention-deficit/hyperactivity disorder among pediatric patients in the United States. *Value in Health, 20*(4), 602–609.

Heilskov Rytter, M. J., Andersen, L. B., Houmann, T., Bilenberg, N., Hvolby, A., Mølgaard, C., et al. (2015). Diet in the treatment of ADHD in children—A systematic review of the literature. *Nordic Journal of Psychiatry, 69*(1), 1–18.

Hemamy, M., Pahlavani, N., Amanollahi, A., Islam, S. M. S., McVicar, J., Askari, G., et al. (2021). The effect of vitamin D and magnesium supplementation on the mental health status of attention-deficit hyperactive children: A randomized controlled trial. *BMC Pediatrics, 21*(1), 178.

Hertz-Picciotto, I., Sass, J. B., Engel, S., Bennett, D. H., Bradman, A., Eskenazi, B., et al. (2018). Organophosphate exposures during pregnancy and child neurodevelopment: Recommendations for essential policy reforms. *PLoS Medicine, 15*(10), e1002671.

Jacobson, M. F., Schardt, D. (1999). *Diet, ADHD & behavior: A quarter-century review [and] a parent's guide to diet, ADHD & behavior.*

Katzman, M. A., Bilkey, T. S., Chokka, P. R., Fallu, A., & Klassen, L. J. (2017). Adult ADHD and comorbid disorders: Clinical implications of a dimensional approach. *BMC Psychiatry, 17*(1), 302.

Kavale, K. A., & Forness, S. R. (1983). Hyperactivity and diet treatment: A meta-analysis of the Feingold hypothesis. *Journal of Learning Disabilities, 16*(6), 324–330.

Khoshbakht, Y., Bidaki, R., & Salehi-Abargouei, A. (2018). Vitamin D status and attention deficit hyperactivity disorder: A systematic review and meta-analysis of observational studies. *Advances in Nutrition, 9*(1), 9–20.

Khoshbakht, Y., Moghtaderi, F., Bidaki, R., Hosseinzadeh, M., & Salehi-Abargouei, A. (2021). The effect of dietary approaches to stop hypertension (DASH) diet on attention-deficit hyperactivity disorder (ADHD) symptoms: A randomized controlled clinical trial. *European Journal of Nutrition, 60*(7), 3647–3658.

Kotsi, E., Kotsi, E., & Perrea, D. N. (2019). Vitamin D levels in children and adolescents with attention-deficit hyperactivity disorder (ADHD): A meta-analysis. *Atten Defic Hyperact Disord, 11*(3), 221–232.

Kumperscak, H. G., Gricar, A., Ülen, I., & Micetic-Turk, D. (2020). A pilot randomized control trial with the probiotic strain lactobacillus rhamnosus GG (LGG) in ADHD: Children and adolescents report better health-related quality of life. *Frontiers in Psychiatry, 11*, 181.

Lange, K. W. (2020). Micronutrients and diets in the treatment of attention-deficit/hyperactivity disorder: Chances and pitfalls. *Frontiers in Psychiatry, 11*, 102.

Lange, K. W., Nakamura, Y., & Reissmann, A. (2022). Diet and food in attention-deficit hyperactivity disorder. *Journal of Future Foods, 2*(2), 112–118.

Lee, K. S., Choi, Y. J., Lim, Y. H., Lee, J. Y., Shin, M. K., Kim, B. N., et al. (2022). Dietary patterns are associated with attention-deficit hyperactivity disorder (ADHD) symptoms among preschoolers in South Korea: A prospective cohort study. *Nutritional Neuroscience, 25*(3), 603–611.

Lopez-Garcia, M., Martinez-Bebia, M., Lopez-Moro, A., Gimenez-Blasi, N., Latorre, J. A., & Mariscal-Arcas, M. (2025). Endocrine disruptors and attention deficit hyperactivity disorder: A systematic review. *Archives of Medical Research, 56*(7), 103260.

Lozoff, B., Castillo, M., Clark, K. M., Smith, J. B., & Sturza, J. (2014). Iron supplementation in infancy contributes to more adaptive behavior at 10 years of age. *The Journal of Nutrition, 144*(6), 838–845.

Maher, B. S., Bitsko, R. H., Claussen, A. H., O'Masta, B., Cerles, A., Holbrook, J. R., et al. (2024). Systematic review and meta-analysis of the relationship between exposure to parental substance use and attention-deficit/hyperactivity disorder in children. *Prevention Science, 25*(Suppl 2), 291–315.

Mahmoud, M. M., El-Mazary, A. A., Maher, R. M., & Saber, M. M. (2011). Zinc, ferritin, magnesium and copper in a group of Egyptian children with attention deficit hyperactivity disorder. *Italian Journal of Pediatrics, 37*, 60.

Mahone, E. M., & Denckla, M. B. (2017). Attention-deficit/hyperactivity disorder: A historical neuropsychological perspective. *Journal of the International Neuropsychological Society, 23*(9–10), 916–929.

Mian, A., Jansen, P. W., Nguyen, A. N., Bowling, A., Renders, C. M., & Voortman, T. (2019). Children's attention-deficit/hyperactivity disorder symptoms predict lower diet quality but not vice versa: Results from bidirectional analyses in a population-based cohort. *The Journal of Nutrition, 149*(4), 642–648.

Millichap, J. G., & Yee, M. M. (2012). The diet factor in attention-deficit/hyperactivity disorder. *Pediatrics, 129*(2), 330–337.

Ng, Q. X., Ho, C. Y. X., Chan, H. W., Yong, B. Z. J., & Yeo, W. S. (2017). Managing childhood and adolescent attention-deficit/hyperactivity disorder (ADHD) with exercise: A systematic review. *Complementary Therapies in Medicine, 34*, 123–128.

Nigg, J. T., Lewis, K., Edinger, T., & Falk, M. (2012). Meta-analysis of attention-deficit/hyperactivity disorder or attention-deficit/hyperactivity disorder symptoms, restriction diet, and synthetic food color additives. *Journal of the American Academy of Child and Adolescent Psychiatry, 51*(1), 86–97.e8.

Nilsen, F. M., & Tulve, N. S. (2020). A systematic review and meta-analysis examining the interrelationships between chemical and non-chemical stressors and inherent characteristics in children with ADHD. *Environmental Research, 180*, 108884.

O'Neal, S. L., & Zheng, W. (2015). Manganese toxicity upon overexposure: A decade in review. *Current Environmental Health Reports, 2*(3), 315–328.

Pelsser, L. M., Frankena, K., Toorman, J., Savelkoul, H. F., Pereira, R. R., & Buitelaar, J. K. (2009). A randomised controlled trial into the effects of food on ADHD. *European Child & Adolescent Psychiatry, 18*(1), 12–19.

Poddar, A., Gaddam, S., Sonnaila, S., Bavaraju, V. S. M., & Agrawal, S. (2025). Unraveling attention-deficit/hyperactivity disorder etiology: Current challenges and future directions in treatment. *NeuroSci, 6*(2), 41.

Ramakrishnan, U., Gonzalez-Casanova, I., Schnaas, L., DiGirolamo, A., Quezada, A. D., Pallo, B. C., et al. (2016). Prenatal supplementation with DHA improves attention at 5 y of age: A randomized controlled trial. *The American Journal of Clinical Nutrition, 104*(4), 1075–1082.

Richardson, E., Seibert, T., & Uli, N. K. (2017). Growth perturbations from stimulant medications and inhaled corticosteroids. *Transl Pediatr, 6*(4), 237–247.

Rojo-Marticella, M., Arija, V., Alda, J., Morales-Hidalgo, P., Esteban-Figuerola, P., & Canals, J. (2022). Do children with attention-deficit/hyperactivity disorder follow a different dietary pattern than that of their control peers? *Nutrients, 14*(6), 1131.

Ryu, S. A., Choi, Y. J., An, H., Kwon, H. J., Ha, M., Hong, Y. C., et al. (2022). Associations between dietary intake and attention deficit hyperactivity disorder (ADHD) scores by repeated measurements in school-age children. *Nutrients, 14*(14), 2919.

Salvat, H., Mohammadi, M. N., Molavi, P., Mostafavi, S. A., Rostami, R., & Salehinejad, M. A. (2022). Nutrient intake, dietary patterns, and anthropometric variables of children with ADHD in comparison to healthy controls: A case-control study. *BMC Pediatrics, 22*(1), 70.

San Mauro Martin, I., Sanz Rojo, S., Garicano Vilar, E., González Cosano, L., Conty de la Campa, R., & Blumenfeld Olivares, J. A. (2021). Lifestyle factors, diet and attention-deficit/hyperactivity disorder in Spanish children—An observational study. *Nutritional Neuroscience, 24*(8), 614–623.

Schab, D. W., & Trinh, N. H. (2004). Do artificial food colors promote hyperactivity in children with hyperactive syndromes? A meta-analysis of double-blind placebo-controlled trials. *Journal of Developmental and Behavioral Pediatrics, 25*(6), 423–434.

Sharma, A., & Couture, J. (2014). A review of the pathophysiology, etiology, and treatment of attention-deficit hyperactivity disorder (ADHD). *The Annals of Pharmacotherapy, 48*(2), 209–225.

Skalny, A. V., Mazaletskaya, A. L., Ajsuvakova, O. P., Bjørklund, G., Skalnaya, M. G., Chao, J. C., et al. (2020). Serum zinc, copper, zinc-to-copper ratio, and other essential elements and minerals in children with attention deficit/hyperactivity disorder (ADHD). *Journal of Trace Elements in Medicine and Biology, 58*, 126445.

Skalny, A. V., Mazaletskaya, A. L., Ajsuvakova, O. P., Bjørklund, G., Skalnaya, M. G., Notova, S. V., et al. (2020). Hair trace element concentrations in autism spectrum disorder (ASD) and attention deficit/hyperactivity disorder (ADHD). *Journal of Trace Elements in Medicine and Biology, 61*, 126539.

Verlaet, A. A., Noriega, D. B., Hermans, N., & Savelkoul, H. F. (2014). Nutrition, immunological mechanisms and dietary immunomodulation in ADHD. *European Child & Adolescent Psychiatry, 23*(7), 519–529.

Vohr, B. R., Poggi Davis, E., Wanke, C. A., & Krebs, N. F. (2017). Neurodevelopment: The impact of nutrition and inflammation during preconception and pregnancy in low-resource settings. *Pediatrics, 139*(Suppl 1), S38–s49.

Wermter, A. K., Laucht, M., Schimmelmann, B. G., Banaschewski, T., Sonuga-Barke, E. J., Rietschel, M., et al. (2010). From nature versus nurture, via nature and nurture, to gene x environment interaction in mental disorders. *European Child & Adolescent Psychiatry, 19*(3), 199–210.

Zhao, X., Page, T. F., Altszuler, A. R., Pelham, W. E., 3rd, Kipp, H., Gnagy, E. M., et al. (2019). Family burden of raising a child with ADHD. *Journal of Abnormal Child Psychology, 47*(8), 1327–1338.

Zulauf, C. A., Sprich, S. E., Safren, S. A., & Wilens, T. E. (2014). The complicated relationship between attention deficit/hyperactivity disorder and substance use disorders. *Current Psychiatry Reports, 16*(3), 436.

Chapter 7
Stress, Anxiety, and Major Depressive Disorder

Abstract

- Definition and Epidemiology: Stress is a physiological and psychological response to internal and external stressors, causing widespread functional and emotional changes. Approximately 35% of individuals report experiencing stress, with slightly higher prevalence in women. Anxiety is a normal adaptive response but becomes pathological when persistent, affecting about 4.05% of the global population. Major depressive disorder (MDD) involves at least one major depressive episode lasting two weeks or more, with a lifetime prevalence of ~12%, and is nearly twice as common in women.
- Etiology: Stress, anxiety, and MDD have multifactorial causes, including genetic, biological, psychological, and environmental factors. Anxiety disorders emerge from genetic vulnerability interacting with stress or trauma, while MDD develops from chronic stress, hormonal fluctuations, early life adversities, and environmental stressors. Dysregulation of the HPA axis, neurotransmitter imbalances, inflammation, and nutritional deficiencies contribute to pathophysiology.
- Nutritional Management: Nutrition plays a key role in supporting brain function and hormonal balance. Healthy dietary patterns, such as the Mediterranean diet, along with probiotics and specific nutrient intake, can reduce stress, anxiety, and depressive symptoms. Adequate energy, protein, complex carbohydrates, omega-3 fatty acids, and essential micronutrients (e.g., vitamins D, C, B6, B12, folate, magnesium, and zinc) are critical.
- Food–Drug Interactions: Antidepressants and anxiolytics may interact with certain foods and alcohol, requiring careful dietary and medication management to avoid adverse effects.

Keywords Stress · Anxiety · Major depressive disorder (MDD) · Dietary management · Micronutrients · Mediterranean diet · Food–drug interactions · Gut–brain axis

M. H. Rouhani et al., *The Healing Plate*, SpringerBriefs in Modern Perspectives on Disability Research, https://doi.org/10.1007/978-981-95-8150-4_7

7.1 Definition and Epidemiology

Stress refers to the physiological and psychological response to internal or external stressors, leading to widespread changes in functional and emotional abilities. Common manifestations include palpitations, sweating, restlessness, and fatigue (Association AP, 2025). Recent surveys indicate that approximately 35% of individuals report experiencing stress, with a slightly higher prevalence among women compared to men (Smith & Wesselbaum, 2025).

Anxiety is a normal adaptive reaction to stress that can enhance attention and performance. Anxiety disorders, however, involve excessive and persistent worry or fear, as defined in the DSM-5, lasting at least 6 months and interfering with daily functioning and abilities (Elizabeth, 2022). Epidemiological data indicate that anxiety disorders affect approximately 4.05% of the global population, equivalent to about 301 million individuals, with women being nearly 1.6 times more frequently affected than men (Javaid et al., 2023).

Major depressive disorder (MDD) is characterized by the occurrence of at least one major depressive episode, lasting a minimum of 2 weeks, and presenting with symptoms such as disability disorders depressed mood, anhedonia, sleep and appetite disturbances, fatigue, impaired concentration, guilt, or suicidal thoughts (Association AP, 2022). MDD is one of the most common psychiatric illnesses, with a lifetime prevalence ranging from 5% to 17% and an average of about 12%. Consistently, its occurrence is nearly twice as frequent in women compared to men (Bains & Abdijadid, 2023).

7.2 Etiology

Stress, anxiety, and MDD share multifactorial etiologies, arising from complex interactions among genetic, biological, psychological, and environmental factors. Stress results from physical, psychological, and environmental stressors that disrupt homeostasis and activate neuroendocrine pathways, primarily the sympathetic-adreno-medullary axis and hypothalamic-pituitary-adrenal (HPA) axis, producing adaptive or maladaptive outcomes (Ketchesin et al., 2017; Mifsud & Reul, 2018). Acute stress is triggered by immediate challenges, whereas chronic or recurrent stress from prolonged exposure to persistent stressors increases vulnerability to anxiety, MDD, and cardiovascular disorders (Ketchesin et al., 2017). Environmental (e.g., noise, pollution), psychological (e.g., work pressure, negative cognition), and physiological (e.g., illness, sleep deprivation, nutritional deficiencies) factors further contribute to stress (Chu et al., 2024).

Anxiety disorders emerge when genetic vulnerability interacts with stress or trauma, leading to heightened vigilance that becomes pervasive and pathological. Early life stressors, including adverse childhood experiences, can "hard-wire" heightened anxiety and panic responses, with additional contributions from medications, substance use, and trauma (Chand & Marwaha, 2023; Raymond & Morrow, 2023).

Similarly, MDD arises from genetic predisposition combined with chronic stress, hormonal fluctuations, early life adversities, and environmental stressors. Dysregulation of the HPA axis, neurotransmitter imbalances, inflammatory processes, and nutritional deficiencies (e.g., omega-3 fatty acids, zinc, and antioxidants) contribute to the pathophysiology (Leonard & Maes, 2012; Sutton et al., 2018). Hormonal changes during menstruation, pregnancy, postpartum, and menopause, as well as low sunlight exposure in seasonal affective disorder, further influence susceptibility (Altemus et al., 2012; Sylvia, 2022).

7.3 Nutritional Management

Nutritional management plays an important role in neurological disorders, including stress, anxiety, and MDD, by supporting brain function and hormones activities (Gibson & Blass, 1999; Singh, 2016; Kris-Etherton et al., 2021). Targeted dietary interventions can enhance neurotransmitter synthesis, support immune function, reduce oxidative stress and inflammation, and regulate gut microbiome balance (Gibson & Blass, 1999; E A., 2024; Gasmi et al., 2022). High-quality dietary patterns along with specific nutrient support have been shown to alleviate depressive symptoms, stabilize stress responses, and reduce anxiety, serving both preventive and therapeutic roles in maintaining mental and neurological health (Singh, 2016; Kris-Etherton et al., 2021).

7.3.1 Nutritional Challenge

In stress, anxiety, and MDD, patients face a range of nutritional challenges that can exacerbate symptoms and complicate clinical management. Chronic stress increases physiological demands for energy, oxygen, and essential micronutrients such as vitamins and minerals (Singh, 2016). This is often accompanied by disrupted appetite and a preference for energy-dense, nutrient-poor foods in individuals with stress, anxiety, and MDD (Alrehaili et al., 2024; Chao et al., 2017; Sedgi et al., 2025; Torres & Nowson, 2007). Such patterns contribute to inflammation and oxidative stress, negatively affecting mental health (Selhub, 2022; Firth et al., 2020). In these conditions, negative alterations in gut microbiota and food intolerances may create a vicious cycle of inflammation and symptom exacerbation (Delgadillo et al., 2025; Nikel et al., 2025).

7.3.2 General Dietary Recommendations

The Mediterranean diet, which emphasizes vegetables, fruits, fish, olive oil, nuts, legumes, and whole grains, reduces inflammation and exerts neurotrophic effects, thereby lowering the risk of stress, anxiety, and MDD (Radkhah et al., 2023). Moreover, probiotics and fermented foods can improve gut microbiota and, via the gut–brain axis, alleviate stress, anxiety, and depressive symptoms (Bravo et al., 2011; Gayathri & Rashmi, 2017; Wastyk et al., 2021). Additionally, some stress-reducing foods that may help alleviate stress include: oranges, spinach, chocolate, coffee, blueberries, broccoli, fish, banana, walnuts, eggs, tea, flax seeds, whole grains, and turkey (Singh, 2016).

7.3.3 Energy and Macronutrients Requirements

Caloric Intake: Stress elevates energy expenditure through increased oxygen use, circulation, and metabolic activity, necessitating adequate caloric intake (Singh, 2016). At the same time, antidepressant and antianxiety medications may promote weight gain (Huh et al., 2025), so energy intake should be carefully monitored to meet metabolic demands without leading to excess weight.

Protein and Carbohydrate: Adequate protein intake is essential for mental health, as amino acids serve as precursors for serotonin, dopamine, and norepinephrine, which are critical for mood regulation (Lieberman, 1999; Hasler, 2010). Tryptophan, phenylalanine, and tyrosine, obtained from foods such as milk, cheese, meat, eggs, chicken, fish, beans, oats, nuts, and whole grains (Gomez-Pinilla, 2012; MacDonald et al., 2020), are particularly important, and deficiencies are associated with anxiety, MDD, and cognitive impairments (W L., 2024). Moreover, theanine is an amino acid that can help reduce stress and anxiety, but effective doses are higher than what is found in a typical cup of tea (Singh, 2016). Human studies indicate that higher total protein intake is linked to lower depressive symptoms (Oh et al., 2020; Migchelbrink et al., 2024). In addition, to enhance the effectiveness of tryptophan-rich meals, it is recommended to pair them with complex carbohydrates while keeping overall protein content moderate. Carbohydrates increase tryptophan availability in the brain, whereas very high protein intake may reduce its uptake (Singh, 2016).

Fat: Healthy fats, particularly omega-3 fatty acids, have demonstrated neuroprotective properties (Dyall, 2015); however, findings on their supplementation in MDD and anxiety remain inconsistent (Nasir & Bloch, 2019).

7.3.4 Micronutrients Requirements and Supplementations

Vitamin C: The maintenance of adrenal health and cortisol homeostasis by vitamin C can indirectly alleviate oxidative stress triggered by chronic stress (Patani et al., 2023).

B vitamins: Among the B vitamins, B6, B12, and folate are especially important for energy metabolism, mood stabilization, and one-carbon pathways (Kennedy, 2016).

Vitamin D: It plays a key role in serotonin regulation (Yu et al., 2023), and levels below 20 ng/mL are associated with a higher risk of psychophysiological disorders, whereas adequate concentrations are linked to reduced risk and potential improvement of conditions such as anxiety and MDD (Silva et al., 2021).

Magnesium and zinc both appear to have therapeutic potential in clinical MDD (Sowa-Kućma et al., 2013), and selenium, copper, manganese, and iodine play important roles in maintaining cognitive health (Li et al., 2025).

7.4 Food–Drug Interactions

Table 7.1 summarizes the major classes of medications used for anxiety and depression, along with representative examples and key considerations regarding food–drug interactions (IA A, 2014; JL MLR, 2020; A SHS, 2023; Parish et al., 2023; R TAM, 2023; RK SSNFKP, 2023; Wilson, 2023; A SDS, 2024; A SJS, 2024; P BCP, 2024; al JTGJFRe, 2025; Lodge, 2025; Media, 2025).

Table 7.1 Commonly prescribed medications for stress, anxiety and major depressive disorder and their food–drug interactions

Drug	Trade name	Food–drug interactions
Antidepressants		
Amitriptyline *(TCA)*	Elavil	**Side effects:** Urinary retention, constipation, xerostomia, dizziness, headache, and somnolence **Avoid:** Alcohol
Sertraline (SSRI)	Zoloft	**Side effects:** Nausea, diarrhea, somnolence, tremor, fatigue **Avoid:** Tryptophan, alcohol, St John's wort, grapefruit juice, herbal products that have antiplatelet effects
Citalopram (SSRI)	Celexa	**Side effects:** Drowsiness, insomnia, dizziness, headache, diaphoresis, nausea, vomiting, xerostomia, constipation, diarrhea **Avoid:** Tryptophan, alcohol, St John's wort, herbal products that have antiplatelet effects
Fluoxetine (SSRI)	Prozac	**Side effects:** Anorexia, dry mouth **Avoid:** Tryptophan, alcohol, herbal products that have antiplatelet effects
Venlafaxine (SNRI)	Effexor	**Side effects:** Headache, sweating, dizziness, nausea, vomiting, or diarrhea **Avoid:** Tryptophan, alcohol, St John's wort, herbal products that have antiplatelet effects
Trazodone	Desyrel	**Side effects:** Headaches, fatigue, dizziness, drowsiness, somnolence, dry mouth **Avoid:** Alcohol, tryptophan, St John's wort, herbs that have antiplatelet effects

(continued)

Table 7.1 (continued)

Drug	Trade name	Food–drug interactions
Bupropion	Wellbutrin	**Side effects:** Dry mouth, constipation, headache, nausea, vomiting, dizziness, sweating**Avoid:** Alcohol, St John's wort
Mirtazapine	Remeron	**Side effects:** Drowsiness, weight gain, xerostomia, increased serum cholesterol, constipation, increase in appetite **Avoid:** Alcohol, tryptophan, St John's wort
Anxiolytics		
Alprazolam	Xanax	**Side effects:** Respiratory depression, respiratory arrest, drowsiness, confusion, headache, syncope, nausea and vomiting, diarrhea, and tremors **Avoid:** Alcohol, caffeine, herbal, and natural products that cause CNS stimulation or sedation
Diazepam	Valium	Similar to alprazolam
Lorazepam	Ativan	Similar to alprazolam
Temazepam	Restoril	Similar to alprazolam
Clonazepam	Restoril	Similar to alprazolam
Buspirone	Buspar	**Side effects:** Ataxia, confusion, dizziness, drowsiness, excitement, headache**Avoid:** Alcohol, St John's wort

Acknowledgments The authors confirm that the content, analysis, and conclusions of this manuscript are their own work. AI-based tools were used solely to assist in improving the clarity and correctness of the English language.

References

A SDS. (2024). *Venlafaxine*. In: StatPearls, editor. Treasure Island (FL): StatPearls Publishing.

A SHS. (2023). *Sertraline: StatPearls*. https://www.ncbi.nlm.nih.gov/books/NBK547689/

A SJS. (2024). *Trazodone: StatPearls*. https://www.ncbi.nlm.nih.gov/books/NBK470560/

al JTGJFRe. (2025). *Mirtazapine*. StatPearls [Internet]. Treasure Island (FL): StatPearls Publishing.

Alexiou, E. (2024). Nutrition in psychiatry: Exploring the mind-body connection. Neuroscience and psychiatry: Open. *Access, 7*(1), 165–167.

Alrehaili, S., Afifi, A. A., Algheshairy, R. M., Bushnaq, T., Alharbi, T. A. F., & Alharbi, H. F. (2024). Prevalence of anhedonia, anxiety, and their impact on food consumption among postgraduate Qassim university students. *Frontiers in Nutrition, 11*, 1445125.

Altemus, M., Neeb, C. C., Davis, A., Occhiogrosso, M., Nguyen, T., & Bleiberg, K. L. (2012). Phenotypic differences between pregnancy-onset and postpartum-onset major depressive disorder. *The Journal of Clinical Psychiatry, 73*(12), e1485–e1491.

Association AP. (2022*). Diagnostic and statistical manual of mental disorders, fifth edition, text revision (DSM-5-TR)*. Text Revision ed. American Psychiatric Association.

Association AP. (2025). *Stress: American psychological association*. https://www.apa.org/topics/stress

Bains, N., & Abdijadid, S. (2023). *Major depressive disorder*. StatPearls [Internet]. Treasure Island (FL): StatPearls Publishing.

Bravo, J. A., Forsythe, P., Chew, M. V., Escaravage, E., Savignac, H. M., Dinan, T. G., et al. (2011). Ingestion of lactobacillus strain regulates emotional behavior and central GABA receptor expression in a mouse via the vagus nerve. *Proceedings of the National Academy of Sciences of the United States of America, 108*(38), 16050–16055.

Chand, S. P., & Marwaha, R. (2023). *Anxiety*. StatPearls [Internet]. Treasure Island (FL): StatPearls Publishing.

Chao, A. M., Jastreboff, A. M., White, M. A., Grilo, C. M., & Sinha, R. (2017). Stress, cortisol, and other appetite-related hormones: Prospective prediction of 6-month changes in food cravings and weight. *Obesity (Silver Spring), 25*(4), 713–720.

Chu, B., Marwaha, K., Sanvictores, T., Awosika, A. O., & Ayers, D. (2024). *Physiology, stress reaction*. StatPearls [Internet]: StatPearls Publishing.

Delgadillo, D. R., Borelli, J. L., Mayer, E. A., Labus, J. S., Cross, M. P., & Pressman, S. D. (2025). Biological, environmental, and psychological stress and the human gut microbiome in healthy adults. *Scientific Reports, 15*(1), 362.

Dyall, S. C. (2015). Long-chain omega-3 fatty acids and the brain: A review of the independent and shared effects of EPA, DPA and DHA. *Frontiers in Aging Neuroscience, 7*, 52.

Elizabeth Arnold, M. (2022). *Anxiety DSM-5 diagnostic criteria and treatment overview: MedCentral*. https://www.medcentral.com/behavioral-mental/anxiety/assessment-diagnosis-adherence-anxiety?utm_source=chatgpt.com

Firth, J., Gangwisch, J. E., Borsini, A., Wootton, R. E., & Mayer, E. A. (2020). Food and mood: how do diet and nutrition affect mental wellbeing? *BMJ, 369*, m2382.

Gasmi, A., Nasreen, A., Menzel, A., Gasmi Benahmed, A., Pivina, L., Noor, S., et al. (2022). Neurotransmitters regulation and food intake: The role of dietary sources in neurotransmission. *Molecules, 28*(1), 210.

Gayathri, D., & Rashmi, B. (2017). Mechanism of development of depression and probiotics as adjuvant therapy for its prevention and management. *Mental Health & Prevention, 5*, 40–51.

Gibson, G. E., & Blass, J. (1999). *Nutrition and functional neurochemistry. Basic neurochemistry: Molecular, cellular and medical aspects* (6th ed., pp. 691–710). Lippincott-Raven.

Gomez-Pinilla, F. (2012). Food and mood; eat yourself happy, healthful element. *Journal of Neurotrauma, 24*, 1587–1595.

Hasler, G. (2010). Pathophysiology of depression: Do we have any solid evidence of interest to clinicians? *World Psychiatry, 9*(3), 155.

Huh, Y., Kim, H. R., & Park, H. S. (2025). Association between antidepressants and antianxiety medications and weight gain in Korean adults aged 19 to 39 years. *The Journal of Clinical Endocrinology and Metabolism, 110*(5), e1499–ee507.

IA A. (2014). *Food-drug interactions and their impact on the pharmacotherapy*. Brno: University of Veterinary and Pharmaceutical Sciences Brno, Faculty of Pharmacy, Department of Human Pharmacology and Toxicology.

Javaid, S. F., Hashim, I. J., Hashim, M. J., Stip, E., Samad, M. A., & Ahbabi, A. A. (2023). Epidemiology of anxiety disorders: Global burden and sociodemographic associations. *Middle East Current Psychiatry, 30*(1), 44.

JL MLR. (2020). *Krause's food & the nutrition care process*. 15th ed. Elsevier.

Kennedy, D. O. (2016). B vitamins and the brain: Mechanisms, dose and efficacy—A review. *Nutrients, 8*(2), 68.

Ketchesin, K. D., Stinnett, G. S., & Seasholtz, A. F. (2017). Corticotropin-releasing hormone-binding protein and stress: From invertebrates to humans. *Stress, 20*(5), 449–464.

Kris-Etherton, P. M., Petersen, K. S., Hibbeln, J. R., Hurley, D., Kolick, V., Peoples, S., et al. (2021). Nutrition and behavioral health disorders: Depression and anxiety. *Nutrition Reviews, 79*(3), 247–260.

Leonard, B., & Maes, M. (2012). Mechanistic explanations how cell-mediated immune activation, inflammation and oxidative and nitrosative stress pathways and their sequels and concomitants play a role in the pathophysiology of unipolar depression. *Neuroscience and Biobehavioral Reviews, 36*(2), 764–785.

Li, H., Yin, Z., Cui, F., Wang, W., & Zhang, D. (2025). The association of dietary essential trace elements and mixture with cognition: A prospective study. *Frontiers in Nutrition, 12*, 1461852.

Lieberman, H. R. (1999). Amino acid and protein requirements: Cognitive performance, stress and brain function. In *The role of protein and amino acids in sustaining and enhancing performance* (pp. 289–307). National Academies Press.

Lodge, B. (2025). *Dangers of mixing amitriptyline and alcohol: Banbury Lodge*. https://www.banburylodge.com/help-guides/dangers-of-mixing-amitriptyline-and-alcohol/

MacDonald, A., Van Wegberg, A., Ahring, K., Beblo, S., Bélanger-Quintana, A., Burlina, A., et al. (2020). PKU dietary handbook to accompany PKU guidelines. *Orphanet Journal of Rare Diseases, 15*(1), 171.

Media, H. (2025). *Bupropion oral tablet: Uses, side effects, and alternatives: Healthline*. https://www.healthline.com/health/drugs/bupropion-oral-tablet#alternatives

Mifsud, K. R., & Reul, J. (2018). Mineralocorticoid and glucocorticoid receptor-mediated control of genomic responses to stress in the brain. *Stress, 21*(5), 389–402.

Migchelbrink, M. M., Kremers, S. H., den Braver, N. R., Groeneveld, L., Elders, P. J., Blom, M. T., et al. (2024). The cross-sectional association between dietary total, animal, and plant-based protein intake and the prevalence and severity of depressive symptoms in Dutch adults with type 2 diabetes: The Hoorn diabetes care system cohort. *Preventive Medicine, 186*, 108065.

Nasir, M., & Bloch, M. H. (2019). Trim the fat: The role of omega-3 fatty acids in psychopharmacology. *Therapeutic Advances in Psychopharmacology, 9*, 2045125319869791.

Nikel, K., Stojko, M., Smolarczyk, J., & Piegza, M. (2025). The impact of gut microbiota on the development of anxiety symptoms—A narrative review. *Nutrients, 17*(6), 933.

Oh, J., Yun, K., Chae, J. H., & Kim, T. S. (2020). Association between macronutrients intake and depression in the United States and South Korea. *Frontiers in Psychiatry, 11*, 207.

P BCP. (2024). *Benzodiazepines*. https://www.ncbi.nlm.nih.gov/books/NBK470159/

Parish, A. L., Gillis, B., & Anthamatten, A. (2023). Pharmacotherapy for depression and anxiety in the primary care setting. *The Journal for Nurse Practitioners, 19*(4), 104556.

Patani, A., Balram, D., Yadav, V. K., Lian, K. Y., Patel, A., & Sahoo, D. K. (2023). Harnessing the power of nutritional antioxidants against adrenal hormone imbalance-associated oxidative stress. *Front Endocrinol (Lausanne)., 14*, 1271521.

R TAM. (2023). *Amitriptyline: StatPearls*. https://www.ncbi.nlm.nih.gov/books/NBK537225/

Radkhah, N., Rasouli, A., Majnouni, A., Eskandari, E., & Parastouei, K. (2023). The effect of Mediterranean diet instructions on depression, anxiety, stress, and anthropometric indices: A randomized, double-blind, controlled clinical trial. *Preventive Medical Reports, 36*, 102469.

Raymond, J. L., & Morrow, K. (2023). *Krause and Mahan's food & the nutrition care process* (16th ed., p. 1280). Elsevier.

RK SSNFKP. (2023). *Citalopram: StatPearls*. https://www.ncbi.nlm.nih.gov/books/NBK482222/

Sedgi, F. M., Hejazi, J., Derakhshi, R., Baghdadi, G., Zarmakhi, M., Hamidi, M., et al. (2025). Investigation of the relationship between food preferences and depression symptoms among undergraduate medical students: A cross-sectional study. *Frontiers in Nutrition, 12*, 1519726.

Selhub, E. (2022). *Nutritional psychiatry: Your brain on food*. Harvard Health Publishing. https://www.health.harvard.edu/blog/nutritional-psychiatry-your-brain-on-food-201511168626

Silva, M. R. M., Barros, W. M. A., Silva, M. L., Silva, J. M. L., Souza, A. P. S., Silva, A. B. J., et al. (2021). Relationship between vitamin D deficiency and psychophysiological variables: A systematic review of the literature. *Clinics, 76*, e3155.

Singh, K. (2016). *Nutrient and stress management*.

Smith, M. D., & Wesselbaum, D. (2025). Global evidence on the prevalence of and risk factors associated with stress. *Journal of Affective Disorders, 374*, 179–183.

Sowa-Kućma, M., Szewczyk, B., Sadlik, K., Piekoszewski, W., Trela, F., Opoka, W., et al. (2013). Zinc, magnesium and NMDA receptor alterations in the hippocampus of suicide victims. *Journal of Affective Disorders, 151*(3), 924–931.

Sutton, L. P., Orlandi, C., Song, C., Oh, W. C., Muntean, B. S., Xie, K., et al. (2018). Orphan receptor GPR158 controls stress-induced depression. *eLife, 7*, e33273.

Sylvia, E.-S. (2022). *Nutrition & diagnosis-related care* (9th ed.). Academy of Nutrition and Dietetics.

Torres, S. J., & Nowson, C. A. (2007). Relationship between stress, eating behavior, and obesity. *Nutrition, 23*(11–12), 887–894.

Wastyk, H. C., Fragiadakis, G. K., Perelman, D., Dahan, D., Merrill, B. D., Yu, F. B., et al. (2021). Gut-microbiota-targeted diets modulate human immune status. *Cell, 184*(16), 4137–53.e14.

White, L. (2024). The advantages of amino acid supplements for cognitive and mental health. *Journal of Nutrition Science, 9*, 275.

Wilson, T., & Tripp, J. (2023). *Buspirone*. StatPearls [Internet]. Treasure Island (FL): StatPearls Publishing.

Yu, X.-L., Li, C.-P., & He, L.-P. (2023). Vitamin D may alleviate irritable bowel syndrome by modulating serotonin synthesis: A hypothesis based on recent literature. *Frontiers in Physiology, 14*, 1152958.

Chapter 8
Dementia and Alzheimer's Disease

Abstract

- Dementia, particularly Alzheimer's disease, causes progressive cognitive decline, severe disability, dependence, and a substantial global healthcare burden.
- Major risk factors include advanced age, APOE gene variants, cardiovascular disease, diabetes, hypertension, midlife obesity, smoking, alcohol, head injury, and deficiencies in thiamine, niacin, and vitamin B12.
- Nutritional challenges manifesting as weight loss, anorexia, impaired taste and smell, swallowing difficulties, behavioral disturbances, and sedative medication effects.
- Diets rich in omega-3 fatty acids, colorful fruits and vegetables, choline sources, nuts, vitamin E, and copper support cognitive function.
- Dietary patterns such as MIND, Mediterranean-DASH, ketogenic, and Keto-Med provide neuroprotective effects.
- Enteral nutrition is indicated for acute or reversible intake reduction, PEG feeding for prolonged needs, while artificial nutrition is discouraged in advanced or terminal dementia.
- Supplementation should address documented deficiencies, focusing on vitamins A, C, D, E, B9, B12, choline, omega-3 fatty acids, and bioactive compounds such as resveratrol, curcumin, and polyphenols.
- Feeding strategies include texture and liquid modification, hand-over-hand guidance, verbal cues, small frequent bites, adaptive utensils, hydration support, and bowel/bladder management.
- Current drug therapy for AD is not curative but offers symptomatic relief; due to the chronic course and older patient age, food–drug interactions are clinically important.

Keywords Dementia · Alzheimer's disease · Neurodevelopmental disorders · Nutrition · Malnutrition · Micronutrients · Enteral nutrition · Parenteral nutrition · Dietary patterns · Food–drug interactions

M. H. Rouhani et al., *The Healing Plate*, SpringerBriefs in Modern Perspectives on Disability Research, https://doi.org/10.1007/978-981-95-8150-4_8

8.1 Definition and Epidemiology

Dementia is a progressive and incapacitating syndrome, widely recognized as a disability disorder, characterized by global cognitive impairment with a decline in memory and at least in one other cognitive domain, such as language, visuospatial, or executive function (Feldman et al., 2008; McKhann et al., 2011). Alzheimer's disease (AD) is the most common type of dementia; other types include vascular dementia, dementia with Lewy bodies, and frontotemporal dementia. As one of the leading disability-related conditions in aging populations, dementia profoundly compromises independence, daily functioning, and social participation. Dementia is currently the seventh leading cause of death and one of the major causes of disability and dependency among older people globally (World Health Organization, 2025). An estimated 7.2 million Americans age 65 and older live with AD today. This number could grow to 13.8 million by 2060, barring the development of medical breakthroughs to prevent or cure AD (Rajan et al., 2021). AD appears to be more prevalent in Western countries and the prevalence is increasing at a faster rate than other chronic diseases. Data from the Framingham Heart Study showed the lifetime risk for AD is about one in ten for men and one in five for women. Total cost of dementia estimates as $781 billion (2025 dollars) (United States Cost of Dementia Research Team, 2025).

8.2 Etiology

An estimated less than 5% of AD cases occur due to rare genetic variants (Seeley & Miller, 2020; Sink & Yaffe, 2014). Recent research identifies a variant of the apolipoprotein E (APOE) gene as a risk factor for AD developing at age 65 or older (late onset). The most proven risk factor for AD is advanced age, with most cases of AD diagnosed at age 65 or older. Other risk factors include, cardiovascular disease, diabetes, hypertension, free radical oxidative damage, long-term/low-dose exposure to pesticides, obesity during midlife, smoking, Down syndrome, and a history of previous head injury (Chen et al., 2017). Heavy drinking and alcohol use disorders are the most important risk factors for dementia, especially for those types of dementia that start before age 65 (Schwarzinger et al., 2018). Possible Nutrition and Metabolic Etiologies of dementia is thiamin, niacin, and vitamin B12 deficiency. Reduced serum thiamine metabolites could be used as an inexpensive and noninvasive diagnostic tool for distinguishing AD from vascular and frontotemporal dementia (Pan et al., 2015; Lu'o'ng & Nguyen, 2011). The pathophysiological changes in the brain associated with AD may begin 20 or more years before the onset of clinical symptoms, providing an opportunity for lifestyle modifications that could slow progression and/or help prevent AD. Protective factors include regular physical activity, maintenance of healthy body weight, social engagement, and cognitive training. Importantly, the role of diet and nutrition in AD prevention and treatment is an active and promising area of research.

8.3 Nutritional Managements

8.3.1 Nutritional Challenges

Dementia leads to gradual cognitive and physiological changes that severely compromise nutrition. Initial symptoms include weight loss, decreased appetite, and impaired smell and taste, which are the main reasons for malnutrition that occur even before diagnosis (Albanese et al., 2013; Gillette Guyonnet et al., 2007; Gillette-Guyonnet et al., 2000; Wang et al., 2021; White et al., 1996). In advanced stages, these symptoms develop into swallowing difficulties, refusal of food, hungry-cue disruption, and caregiver issues (Unsal et al., 2023). Moreover, behavioral disturbances such as agitation markedly elevate energy expenditure, while the use of sedative medications may profoundly suppress appetite and significantly reduce dietary intake (Aliani et al., 2013; Chang & Roberts, 2008; Chouinard et al., 1998; Cipriani et al., 2016; Doorduijn et al., 2020; Keller et al., 2006; Langmore et al., 2002; Lechowski et al., 2008; Silva et al., 2013; Watson & Deary, 1994; Aselage & Amella, 2010; Alagiakrishnan et al., 2013). Also, age-related comorbidities such as chewing problems, dehydration, depression, and continence issues serve to limit the consumption of food and fluids (Agarwal et al., 2013; Dent et al., 2023; Volkert et al., 2019). Over 95% of AD patients are reported to be malnourished or at risk (Tombini et al., 2016). Inadequate intake precipitates sarcopenia, frailty, and elevated mortality, while nutrient deficiencies may accelerate cognitive decline, creating a vicious cycle (Unsal et al., 2023; Waite et al., 2021; Faxén-Irving et al., 2005).

8.3.2 General Dietary Recommendations

A targeted nutritional strategy for dementia prevention and management advocates a healthy diet rich in specific anti-inflammatory and antioxidant compounds from whole food sources. Key recommendations include prioritizing oily fish (salmon, halibut, tuna) for omega-3 fatty acids as primary omega-3 sources over supplements, incorporating flavanol-rich foods like coffee and cocoa, ensuring adequate B vitamins intakes from leafy greens and broccoli, obtaining choline from soybeans and eggs, and emphasizing deeply colored fruits (blueberries, cranberries, strawberries, berries, citrus), and vegetables (spinach, kale) for their phytonutrient content. Additionally, sources of copper (liver, kidney, oysters, nuts, beans, cocoa, eggs, prunes, potatoes), and vitamin E (nuts, dressings) should be emphasized included (Valls-Pedret et al., 2012). Notably, junk food consumption exerts deleterious effects on AD (Hill et al., 2018). While certain foods traditionally deemed harmful (e.g., eggs, red meat) have undergone partial rehabilitated, excessive saturated fat intake remains detrimental (Solfrizzi & Panza, 2014).

The MIND Diet or Mediterranean-DASH intervention (Carbohydrates: 45–55%; Protein: 15–20%; Total fat: 25–30%; and Sodium intake: 2400 mg/d) (Asemi et al.,

2013) for neurodegenerative delay has been found to substantially slow cognitive decline with aging and the risk of AD (Morris et al., 2015; Morris et al., 2015b). Also, ketogenic diet (KD) has beneficial effects on improving cognitive performance in older adults with AD. The level and duration of ketosis affect the improvement of cognitive outcomes (Rusek et al., 2019). Ketogenic diets are low-carbohydrate, high-fat, moderate-protein diets that typically provide about 80% of calories from fat, 15% from protein, and 5% from carbohydrates (Veech, 2004). Medium-chain triglyceride (MCT) oil, a major lipid component in KD, may promote ketogenesis and maintain mitochondrial function, in conjunctive therapy for AD patients (Takeishi et al., 2021; Hu Yang et al., 2015). Another intervention is the Keto-Mediet, which combines the benefits of a KD and a Mediterranean diet in a model that is rich in various types of vitamins, substitutes coconut oil for saturated animal fats, and limits glucose intake (Perng et al., 2017).

8.3.3 Energy Requirements

Energy needs must be individualized based on age, sex, and physical activity levels. Notably, patients who are "wanderers" or highly active require a high-calorie intake (approximately 35 kcal/kg) and sufficient protein to prevent catabolism. The goal is to maintain a reasonable body weight, typically within a BMI range of 22–27 kg/m^2. Several interventions using liquid supplements have demonstrated efficacy in promoting weight gain and overall nutritional intake in patients with AD (Pivi et al., 2011; Vicente de Sousa et al., 2017). Supplementation have been shown to be least effective in individuals with the lowest BMIs; thus, it may be most helpful to institute interventions early when weight loss begins (Smith & Greenwood, 2008; Dorner et al., 2010).

8.3.4 Enteral and Parenteral Nutrition

Each decision for or against (par) enteral nutrition and hydration for persons with dementia shall be made on an individual basis with respect to the patient's clinical situation, general prognosis, and preferences. Temporary feeding through the gastrointestinal tract might be considered in moderate to mild dementia if a short, severe oral intake drop (<50% of energy requirements for >7 days) brought about by a potentially reversible cause has been diagnosed, even when adequate support and oral supplementation have been provided. Nasogastric feeding is the initial option; however, if less feeding is expected for over 2 weeks or if feeding through a nasogastric tube is not tolerated, a percutaneous endoscopic gastrostomy (PEG) should be considered. Low-profile PEG tubes ("buttons") are preferred for individuals with dementia, at risk of pulling out protruding tubes.

There is no valuable outcome with tube feeding when reduced intake reflects disease progression. If partial oral intake resumes, discontinuation of EN should be evaluated. EN/PN and parenteral fluids are not recommended in terminal dementia due to increased risks such as aspiration pneumonia, diarrhea and gastrointestinal discomfort, pressure ulcers (EN), bloodstream infections (PN), and also discomfort from secretions or pulmonary edema (Sampson et al., 2009; Comerlato et al., 2021). The American Geriatrics Society does not recommend feeding tubes for advanced dementia adults and instead suggests assisted feeding, person-centered approaches, and environmental adjustments to maximize oral intake. Monitoring of the weight and routine malnutrition screening are the two basic parts of the process. Artificial nutrition is suitable only in mild to moderate dementia with acute, reversible conditions, not in severe or terminal stages.

8.3.5 Targeted Nutrients and Supplements

Micronutrient supplementation should not be routinely offered to individuals with dementia unless a documented deficiency is present. In such cases, targeted supplementation at physiological (not mega) doses is recommended, with careful consideration of potential toxicity. While the benefit of vitamin supplementation in AD remains debated, some evidence suggests potential effectiveness in specific contexts.

- Vitamin A: The main functions of this vitamin include neurodevelopment, nervous system regeneration, and neurodegenerative processes management, such as AD despite very limited clinical evidence for supplementation (Biyong et al., 2021; Su et al., 2022).
- Vitamin C (500–1000 mg/day): May reduce plasma homocysteine and improve cognitive outcomes in AD (Asemi et al., 2013).
- Vitamin E: Due to its antioxidant properties, has been proposed for AD management, though clinical trials have reported inconsistent outcomes. Meanwhile, adequate intake through diet, rather than supplements, appears beneficial in slowing disease progression (Morris et al., 2002).
- Vitamin D: Studies have demonstrated a correlation between high levels of circulating 25(OH)D (≥50 nmol/L) and a lower incidence of dementia and AD, as well as slower rates of cognitive decline, indicating that vitamin D may play a neuroprotective role (Feart et al., 2017; Geng et al., 2022).
- Folate (Vitamin B9): Folic acid supplementation could improve cognitive function in AD (Chen et al., 2016a; Chen et al., 2016b; Luchsinger et al., 2007). Intakes equal to or more than the RDA (400 μg/day) has been linked with a reduction in AD risk through lowering homocysteine levels (Corrada et al., 2005). Supplementation with 1 mg/day folate in combination with cholinesterase inhibitors led to the functional outcomes' improvements (Connelly et al., 2008).
- Vitamin B12 (Cobalamin): Low vitamin B12 is associated with cognitive impairment and dementia.
- n-3 Fatty acids: High baseline plasma n-3 fatty acid (FA) level is absolutely necessary to achieve the results of high-dose B vitamin therapy,

- Bioactive compounds (such as pentacyclic triterpenoids (Szuster-Ciesielska et al., 2011), marine phenolics (Lee & Jeon, 2015), α-lipoic acid (Udupa et al., 2012), resveratrol (Szkudelski & Szkudelska, 2015; Kulashekar et al., 2018), curcumin (Thota et al., 2020; Lee et al., 2014; Reddy et al., 2018), gallic acid (Jia et al., 2017; Lupaescu et al., 2022), anthocyanins (Khan et al., 2021), luteolin (Wagle et al., 2019), hesperetin (Lai et al., 2022), genistein (Viña et al., 2022), Boswellia serrata gum extract (Gomaa et al., 2021), mangiferin (Feng et al., 2019), lycopene (Ratto et al., 2021), epigallocatechin-3-gallate, genistein, and flavonoids (Ben Hmidene et al., 2017) have been assessed to decrease risk of AD. Further clinical trials are necessary to establish the efficacy of these components in dementia management.

8.3.6 *Other Considerations*

- Iron accumulation in the brain is one of the hallmarks of AD. Also, clinical evidence suggests that a high zinc supply may lead to a lack of copper, thus giving rise to neurological injury that can be irreversible even after copper repletion (Afrin, 2010).
- Emerging evidence confirms the oral–gut–brain axis as one of the main regulators of neurocognitive decline (Mohajeri et al., 2018). A symbiotic diet model that combines prebiotic fibers, probiotic-rich fermented foods, and anti-inflammatory, plant-based polyphenols appear to be the mainstay of intervention.
- Advanced glycation end products (AGEs) are implicated in the initiation and progression of Alzheimer-type dementia (Lovestone & Smith, 2014).

8.3.7 *Practical Feeding and Care Guidelines*

- Texture and liquid modifications should be applied to reduce aspiration and improve intake.
- Support of eating-related behavior: hand guidance, verbal cues, serve one food at a time, take small bites, frequent snacks, soothing pre-meal music.
- Maximize food intake during lunch when cognition is usually best.
- Simple and stable environment: an uncluttered table, plain-colored plates, one utensil per meal, and the routine schedules kept.
- Self-feeding encouraged; adaptive utensils (special spoons, mugs) provided when needed.
- Prevent constipation and dehydration; maintain regular bowel/bladder routines.

8.4 Food–Drug Interactions

Drug therapy is not currently able to cure AD, but several pharmacological agents are approved to provide symptomatic benefit and to manage cognitive and behavioral disturbances associated with the condition. Given the chronic nature of AD and the older age of most patients, food–drug interactions represent an important consideration in clinical management. The most common medication that are used in dementia disorder along with their food–drug interaction illustrated is in Table 8.1.

Table 8.1 Commonly prescribed medications for dementia disorder and their food–drug interactions

Drug	Trade name	Food–drug interactions
NMDA receptor antagonist		
Memantine	Namenda®	**Side effects:** Constipation, weight gain **Avoid** alcohol, excessive alkaline-forming foods
Cholinesterase inhibitor		
Galantamine	Razadyne	**Side effects:** Weight loss, nausea, vomiting, loss of appetite, and increased frequency of bowel movements. **Avoid:** Alcohol
Donepezil	Aricept	**Side effects:** Nausea, vomiting, loss of appetite, and increased frequency of bowel movements **Avoid:** Alcohol
Rivastigmine	Exelon	**Side effects:** Nausea, vomiting, loss of appetite, and increased frequency of bowel movements. **Avoid: –**
Benzgalantamine	Zunveyl	**Side effects:** Vomiting, diarrhea, loss of appetite, and nausea **Avoid:** Alcohol
Antipsychotic		
Olanzapine	Zyprexa	**Side effects:** Large weight gain, increased appetite **Avoid:** Alcohol, grapefruit
Quetiapine	Seroquel	**Side effects:** Small weight gain, increased appetite **Avoid:** Alcohol, grapefruit
Risperidone	Risperdal	**Side effects:** Moderate weight gain, hypokalemia, increased appetite, diarrhea, and constipation **Avoid**: Alcohol
Brexpiprazole	Rexulti	**Side effects:** Weight gain, constipation, diarrhea, increased appetite **Avoid**: Alcohol, grapefruit juice
Haloperidol	Haldol	**Side effects:** Constipation, xerostomia, and loss of appetite **Avoid**: Alcohol

(continued)

Table 8.1 (continued)

Drug	Trade name	Food–drug interactions
Orexin receptor antagonist		
Suvorexant	Belsomra	**Side effects:** Xerostomia, diarrhea **Avoid**: Grapefruit, St. John's wort
Miscellaneous central nervous system agents		
Ergoloid mesylates	Hydergine	**Side effects:** Loss of appetite, upset stomach, and vomiting **Avoid:** Alcohol, grapefruit
Antidepressants		
Citalopram	Celexa	**Side effects:** Xerostomia **Avoid:** St John's wort and alcohol
Escitalopram	Lexapro	**Side effects:** Xerostomia, diarrhea **Avoid:** St John's wort and alcohol
Fluoxetine	Prozac	**Side effects:** Anorexia, hypokalemia **Avoid:** Alcohol
Paroxetine	Paxil	**Side effects:** Increase appetite **Avoid:** Alcohol, St John's wort
Sertraline	Zoloff	**Side effects:** Xerostomia, diarrhea **Avoid:** Alcohol, St John's wort, and grapefruit or grapefruit juice

Acknowledgments The authors confirm that the content, analysis, and conclusions of this manuscript are their own work. AI-based tools were used solely to assist in improving the clarity and correctness of the English language.

References

Afrin, L. B. (2010). Fatal copper deficiency from excessive use of zinc-based denture adhesive. *The American Journal of the Medical Sciences, 340*(2), 164–168.

Agarwal, E., Miller, M., Yaxley, A., & Isenring, E. (2013). Malnutrition in the elderly: A narrative review. *Maturitas, 76*(4), 296–302.

Alagiakrishnan, K., Bhanji, R. A., & Kurian, M. (2013). Evaluation and management of oropharyngeal dysphagia in different types of dementia: A systematic review. *Archives of Gerontology and Geriatrics, 56*(1), 1–9.

Albanese, E., Taylor, C., Siervo, M., Stewart, R., Prince, M. J., & Acosta, D. (2013). Dementia severity and weight loss: A comparison across eight cohorts. The 10/66 study. *Alzheimers Dement, 9*(6), 649–656.

Aliani, M., Udenigwe, C. C., Girgih, A. T., Pownall, T. L., Bugera, J. L., & Eskin, M. N. (2013). Aroma and taste perceptions with Alzheimer disease and stroke. *Critical Reviews in Food Science and Nutrition, 53*(7), 760–769.

Aselage, M. B., & Amella, E. J. (2010). An evolutionary analysis of mealtime difficulties in older adults with dementia. *Journal of Clinical Nursing, 19*(1–2), 33–41.

Asemi, Z., Tabassi, Z., Samimi, M., Fahiminejad, T., & Esmaillzadeh, A. (2013). Favourable effects of the dietary approaches to stop hypertension diet on glucose tolerance and lipid profiles in gestational diabetes: A randomised clinical trial. *The British Journal of Nutrition, 109*(11), 2024–2030.

Ben Hmidene, A., Hanaki, M., Murakami, K., Irie, K., Isoda, H., & Shigemori, H. (2017). Inhibitory activities of antioxidant flavonoids from Tamarix gallica on amyloid aggregation related to Alzheimer's and type 2 diabetes diseases. *Biological & Pharmaceutical Bulletin, 40*(2), 238–241.

Biyong, E. F., Tremblay, C., Leclerc, M., Caron, V., Alfos, S., Helbling, J. C., et al. (2021). Role of retinoid X receptors (RXRs) and dietary vitamin a in Alzheimer's disease: Evidence from clinicopathological and preclinical studies. *Neurobiology of Disease, 161*, 105542.

Chang, C. C., & Roberts, B. L. (2008). Feeding difficulty in older adults with dementia. *Journal of Clinical Nursing, 17*(17), 2266–2274.

Chen, H., Kwong, J. C., Copes, R., Tu, K., Villeneuve, P. J., van Donkelaar, A., et al. (2017). Living near major roads and the incidence of dementia, Parkinson's disease, and multiple sclerosis: A population-based cohort study. *Lancet, 389*(10070), 718–726.

Chen, H., Liu, S., Ji, L., Wu, T., Ji, Y., Zhou, Y., et al. (2016a). Folic acid supplementation mitigates Alzheimer's disease by reducing inflammation: A randomized controlled trial. *Mediators of Inflammation, 2016*, 5912146.

Chen, H., Liu, S., Ji, L., et al. (2016b). Folic acid supplementation mitigates Alzheimer's disease by reducing inflammation: A randomized controlled trial. *Mediators of Inflammation, 2016*, 5912146. https://doi.org/10.1155/2016/5912146

Chouinard, J., Lavigne, E., & Villeneuve, C. (1998). Weight loss, dysphagia, and outcome in advanced dementia. *Dysphagia, 13*(3), 151–155.

Cipriani, G., Carlesi, C., Lucetti, C., Danti, S., & Nuti, A. (2016). Eating Behaviors and dietary changes in patients with dementia. *American Journal of Alzheimer's Disease and Other Dementias, 31*(8), 706–716.

Comerlato, P. H., Stefani, J., & Viana, L. V. (2021). Mortality and overall and specific infection complication rates in patients who receive parenteral nutrition: Systematic review and meta-analysis with trial sequential analysis. *The American Journal of Clinical Nutrition, 114*(4), 1535–1545.

Connelly, P. J., Prentice, N. P., Cousland, G., et al. (2008). A randomized double-blind placebo-controlled trial of folic acid supplementation of cholinesterase inhibitors in Alzheimer's disease. *International Journal of Geriatric Psychiatry, 23*, 155–160.

Corrada, M. M., Kawas, C. H., Hallfrisch, J., et al. (2005). Reduced risk of Alzheimer's disease with high folate intake: The Baltimore longitudinal study of aging. *Alzheimers Dement, 1*, 11–18.

Dent, E., Wright, O. R. L., Woo, J., & Hoogendijk, E. O. (2023). Malnutrition in older adults. *Lancet, 401*(10380), 951–966.

Doorduijn, A. S., de van der Schueren, M. A. E., van de Rest, O., de Leeuw, F. A., Fieldhouse, J. L. P., Kester, M. I., et al. (2020). Olfactory and gustatory functioning and food preferences of patients with Alzheimer's disease and mild cognitive impairment compared to controls: The NUDAD project. *Journal of Neurology, 267*(1), 144–152.

Dorner, B., Friedrich, E. K., & Posthauer, M. E. (2010). Position of the American dietetic association: Individualized nutrition approaches for older adults in health care communities. *Journal of the American Dietetic Association, 110*(10), 1549–1553.

Faxén-Irving, G., Basun, H., & Cederholm, T. (2005). Nutritional and cognitive relationships and long-term mortality in patients with various dementia disorders. *Age and Ageing, 34*(2), 136–141.

Feart, C., Helmer, C., Merle, B., Herrmann, F. R., Annweiler, C., Dartigues, J. F., et al. (2017). Associations of lower vitamin D concentrations with cognitive decline and long-term risk of dementia and Alzheimer's disease in older adults. *Alzheimer's & Dementia, 13*(11), 1207–1216.

Feldman, H. H., Jacova, C., Robillard, A., Garcia, A., Chow, T., Borrie, M., et al. (2008). Diagnosis and treatment of dementia: 2. Diagnosis. *CMAJ, 178*(7), 825–836.

Feng, S.-T., Wang, Z.-Z., Yuan, Y.-H., Sun, H.-M., Chen, N.-H., & Zhang, Y. (2019). Mangiferin: A multipotent natural product preventing neurodegeneration in Alzheimer's and Parkinson's disease models. *Pharmacological Research, 146*, 104336.

Geng, T., Lu, Q., Wan, Z., Guo, J., Liu, L., Pan, A., et al. (2022). Association of serum 25-hydroxyvitamin D concentrations with risk of dementia among individuals with type 2 diabetes: A cohort study in the UK biobank. *PLoS Medicine, 19*(1), e1003906.

Gillette Guyonnet, S., Abellan Van Kan, G., Alix, E., Andrieu, S., Belmin, J., Berrut, G., et al. (2007). IANA (international academy on nutrition and aging) expert group: Weight loss and Alzheimer's disease. *The Journal of Nutrition, Health & Aging, 11*(1), 38–48.

Gillette-Guyonnet, S., Nourhashemi, F., Andrieu, S., de Glisezinski, I., Ousset, P. J., Riviere, D., et al. (2000). Weight loss in Alzheimer disease. *The American Journal of Clinical Nutrition, 71*(2), 637s–642s.

Gomaa, A. A., Farghaly, H. A., Abdel-Wadood, Y. A., & Gomaa, G. A. (2021). Potential therapeutic effects of boswellic acids/Boswellia serrata extract in the prevention and therapy of type 2 diabetes and Alzheimer's disease. *Naunyn-Schmiedeberg's Archives of Pharmacology, 394*(11), 2167–2185.

Hill, E., Clifton, P., Goodwill, A. M., Dennerstein, L., Campbell, S., & Szoeke, C. (2018). Dietary patterns and β-amyloid deposition in aging Australian women. *Alzheimers Dement (N Y)., 4*, 535–541.

Hu Yang, I., De la Rubia Ortí, J. E., Selvi Sabater, P., Sancho Castillo, S., Rochina, M. J., Manresa Ramón, N., et al. (2015). Coconut oil: Non-alternative drug treatment against ALZHEIMER'S disease. *Nutrición Hospitalaria, 32*(6), 2822–2827.

Jia, J. J., Zeng, X. S., Song, X. Q., Zhang, P. P., & Chen, L. (2017). Diabetes mellitus and Alzheimer's disease: The protection of Epigallocatechin-3-gallate in Streptozotocin injection-induced models. *Frontiers in Pharmacology, 8*, 834.

Keller, H. H., Edward, H. G., & Cook, C. (2006). Mealtime experiences of families with dementia. *American Journal of Alzheimer's Disease and Other Dementias, 21*(6), 431–438.

Khan, M. S., Ikram, M., Park, T. J., & Kim, M. O. (2021). Pathology, risk factors, and oxidative damage related to type 2 diabetes-mediated Alzheimer's disease and the rescuing effects of the potent antioxidant anthocyanin. *Oxidative Medicine and Cellular Longevity, 2021*, 4051207.

Kulashekar, M., Stom, S. M., & Peuler, J. D. (2018). Resveratrol's potential in the adjunctive Management of Cardiovascular Disease, obesity, diabetes, Alzheimer disease, and cancer. *The Journal of the American Osteopathic Association, 118*(9), 596–605.

Lai, M. C., Liu, W. Y., Liou, S. S., & Liu, I. M. (2022). The citrus flavonoid Hesperetin encounters diabetes-mediated Alzheimer-type Neuropathologic changes through relieving advanced glycation end-products inducing endoplasmic reticulum stress. *Nutrients, 14*(4), 745.

Langmore, S. E., Skarupski, K. A., Park, P. S., & Fries, B. E. (2002). Predictors of aspiration pneumonia in nursing home residents. *Dysphagia, 17*(4), 298–307.

Lechowski, L., de Stampa, M., Denis, B., Tortrat, D., Chassagne, P., Robert, P., et al. (2008). Patterns of loss of abilities in instrumental activities of daily living in Alzheimer's disease: The REAL cohort study. *Dementia and Geriatric Cognitive Disorders, 25*(1), 46–53.

Lee, M. S., Wahlqvist, M. L., Chou, Y. C., Fang, W. H., Lee, J. T., Kuan, J. C., et al. (2014). Turmeric improves post-prandial working memory in pre-diabetes independent of insulin. *Asia Pacific Journal of Clinical Nutrition, 23*(4), 581–591.

Lee, S. H., & Jeon, Y. J. (2015). Efficacy and safety of a dieckol-rich extract (AG-dieckol) of brown algae, Ecklonia cava, in pre-diabetic individuals: A double-blind, randomized, placebo-controlled clinical trial. *Food & Function, 6*(3), 853–858.

Lovestone, S., & Smith, U. (2014). Advanced glycation end products, dementia, and diabetes. *Proceedings of the National Academy of Sciences of the United States of America, 111*(13), 4743–4744.

Lu'o'ng, K. V., & Nguyen, L. T. (2011). Role of thiamine in Alzheimer's disease. *American Journal of Alzheimer's Disease and Other Dementias, 26*, 588–598.

Luchsinger, J. A., Tanx, M. X., Miller, J., et al. (2007). Relation of higher folate intake to lower risk of Alzheimer disease in the elderly. *Archives of Neurology, 64*, 86–92.

Lupaescu, A. V., Iavorschi, M., & Covasa, M. (2022). The use of bioactive compounds in Hyperglycemia- and amyloid fibrils-induced toxicity in type 2 diabetes and Alzheimer's disease. *Pharmaceutics., 14*(2), 235.

McKhann, G. M., Knopman, D. S., Chertkow, H., Hyman, B. T., Jack, C. R., Jr., Kawas, C. H., et al. (2011). The diagnosis of dementia due to Alzheimer's disease: Recommendations from the National Institute on Aging-Alzheimer's Association workgroups on diagnostic guidelines for Alzheimer's disease. *Alzheimers Dement, 7*(3), 263–269.

Mohajeri, M. H., La Fata, G., Steinert, R. E., et al. (2018). Relationship between the gut microbiome and brain function. *Nutrition Reviews, 76*(7), 481–496.

Morris, M. C., Evans, D. A., Bienias, J. L., et al. (2002). Dietary intake of antioxidant nutrients and the risk of incident Alzheimer disease in a biracial community study. *JAMA, 287*(24), 3230–3237.

Morris, M. C., Tangney, C. C., Wang, Y., et al. (2015). MIND diet slows cognitive decline with aging. *Alzheimers Dement, 11*, 1015–1022.

Morris, M. C., Tangney, C. C., Wang, Y., et al. (2015b). MIND diet associated with reduced incidence of Alzheimer's disease. *Alzheimers Dement, 11*(9), 1007–1014.

Pan, X., Fei, G., Lu, J., et al. (2015). Measurement of blood thiamine metabolites for Alzheimer's disease diagnosis. *eBioMedicine, 26*(3), 155–162.

Perng, B. C., Chen, M., Perng, J. C., & Jambazian, P. (2017). A keto-Mediet approach with coconut substitution and exercise may delay the onset of Alzheimer's disease among middle-aged. *The Journal of Prevention of Alzheimer's Disease, 4*(1), 51–57.

Pivi, G. A., da Silva, R. V., Juliano, Y., Novo, N. F., Okamoto, I. H., Brant, C. Q., et al. (2011). A prospective study of nutrition education and oral nutritional supplementation in patients with Alzheimer's disease. *Nutrition Journal, 10*, 98.

Rajan, K. B., Weuve, J., Barnes, L. L., McAninch, E. A., Wilson, R. S., & Evans, D. A. (2021). Population estimate of people with clinical Alzheimer's disease and mild cognitive impairment in the United States (2020–2060). *Alzheimers Dement, 17*(12), 1966–1975.

Ratto, F., Franchini, F., Musicco, M., Caruso, G., & Di Santo, S. (2021). A narrative review on the potential of tomato and lycopene for the prevention of Alzheimer's disease and other dementias. *Critical Reviews in Food Science and Nutrition, 62*(18), 4970–4981.

Reddy, P. H., Manczak, M., Yin, X., et al. (2018). Protective effects of Indian spice curcumin against amyloid Beta in Alzheimer's disease. *Journal of Alzheimer's Disease, 61*(3), 843–866.

Rusek, M., Pluta, R., Ułamek-Kozioł, M., & Czuczwar, S. J. (2019). Ketogenic Diet in Alzheimer's Disease. *International Journal of Molecular Sciences, 20*(16), 3892.

Sampson, E. L., Candy, B., & Jones, L. (2009). Enteral tube feeding for older people with advanced dementia. *Cochrane Database of Systematic Reviews, 2009*(2), Cd007209.

Schwarzinger, M., Pollock, B. G., Hasan, O. S. M., Dufouil, C., & Rehm, J. (2018). Contribution of alcohol use disorders to the burden of dementia in France 2008–13: A nationwide retrospective cohort study. *The Lancet Public Health, 3*(3), e124–ee32.

Seeley, W. W., & Miller, B. L. (2020). Alzheimer's Disease. In Jameson J, Fauci AS, Kasper DL, Hauser SL, Longo DL, & Loscalzo J. (Eds.), *Harrison's principles of internal medicine*. McGraw-Hill. Retrieved November 26, 2018, from http://accessmedicine.mhmedical.com/content.aspx?bookid=2129§ionid=192532255

Silva, P., Kergoat, M. J., & Shatenstein, B. (2013). Challenges in managing the diet of older adults with early-stage Alzheimer dementia: A caregiver perspective. *The Journal of Nutrition, Health & Aging, 17*(2), 142–147.

Sink, K. M., & Yaffe, K. (2014). Cognitive impairment & dementia. In B. A. Williams, A. Chang, C. Ahalt, H. Chen, R. Conant, C. Landefeld, C. Ritchie, & M. Yukawa (Eds.), *Current Diagnosis & Treatment: Geriatrics* (2nd ed.). McGraw-Hill. Retrieved September 11, 2018, from http://accessmedicine.mhmedical.com.proxy.lib.ohio-state.edu/content.aspx?bookid=953&sec-tionid=53375646

Smith, K. L., & Greenwood, C. E. (2008). Weight loss and nutritional considerations in Alzheimer disease. *Journal of Nutrition for the Elderly, 27*(3–4), 381–403.

Solfrizzi, V., & Panza, F. (2014). Mediterranean diet and cognitive decline. A lesson from the whole-diet approach: What challenges lie ahead? *Journal of Alzheimer's Disease, 39*(2), 283–286.

Su, L., He, J., Liu, Z., Wu, S., Chen, P., Li, K., et al. (2022). Dietary Total vitamin a, β-carotene, and retinol intake and the risk of diabetes in Chinese adults with plant-based diets. *The Journal of Clinical Endocrinology and Metabolism, 107*(10), e4106–e4e14.

Szkudelski, T., & Szkudelska, K. (2015). Resveratrol and diabetes: From animal to human studies. *Biochimica et Biophysica Acta (BBA)—Molecular Basis of Disease, 1852*(6), 1145–1154.

Szuster-Ciesielska, A., Plewka, K., Daniluk, J., & Kandefer-Szerszeń, M. (2011). Betulin and betulinic acid attenuate ethanol-induced liver stellate cell activation by inhibiting reactive oxygen species (ROS), cytokine (TNF-α, TGF-β) production and by influencing intracellular signaling. *Toxicology, 280*(3), 152–163.

Takeishi, J., Tatewaki, Y., Nakase, T., Takano, Y., Tomita, N., Yamamoto, S., et al. (2021). Alzheimer's disease and type 2 diabetes mellitus: The use of MCT oil and a ketogenic diet. *International Journal of Molecular Sciences, 22*(22), 12310.

Thota, R. N., Rosato, J. I., Dias, C. B., Burrows, T. L., Martins, R. N., & Garg, M. L. (2020). Dietary supplementation with curcumin reduce circulating levels of glycogen synthase kinase-3β and islet amyloid polypeptide in adults with high risk of type 2 diabetes and Alzheimer's disease. *Nutrients, 12*(4), 1032.

Tombini, M., Sicari, M., Pellegrino, G., Ursini, F., Insardá, P., & Di Lazzaro, V. (2016). Nutritional status of patients with Alzheimer's disease and their caregivers. *Journal of Alzheimer's Disease, 54*(4), 1619–1627.

Udupa, A. S., Nahar, P. S., Shah, S. H., Kshirsagar, M. J., & Ghongane, B. B. (2012). Study of comparative effects of antioxidants on insulin sensitivity in type 2 diabetes mellitus. *Journal of Clinical and Diagnostic Research, 6*(9), 1469–1473.

United States Cost of Dementia Research Team. (2025, April 23). *The cost of dementia in 2025 [Internet]*. Retrieved August 26, 2025, from https://schaeffer.usc.edu/research/the-cost-of-dementia-in-2025/

Unsal, P., Guner, M., Ozsurekci, C., Balli, N., Bas, A. O., Ozturk, Y., et al. (2023). Prevalence of nutrition disorders and nutrition-related conditions in older patients with Alzheimer's disease. *Nutrition in Clinical Practice, 38*(5), 1142–1153.

Valls-Pedret, C., Lamuela-Raventós, R. M., Medina-Remón, A., et al. (2012). Polyphenol-rich foods in the Mediterranean diet are associated with better cognitive function in elderly subjects at high cardiovascular risk. *Journal of Alzheimer's Disease, 29*, 773–782.

Veech, R. L. (2004). The therapeutic implications of ketone bodies: The effects of ketone bodies in pathological conditions: Ketosis, ketogenic diet, redox states, insulin resistance, and mitochondrial metabolism. *Prostaglandins, Leukotrienes, and Essential Fatty Acids, 70*(3), 309–319.

Vicente de Sousa, O., Soares Guerra, R., Sousa, A. S., Pais Henriques, B., Pereira Monteiro, A., & Amaral, T. F. (2017). Impact of nutritional supplementation and a psychomotor program on patients with Alzheimer's disease. *American Journal of Alzheimer's Disease and Other Dementias, 32*(6), 329–341.

Viña, J., Escudero, J., Baquero, M., Cebrián, M., Carbonell-Asíns, J. A., Muñoz, J. E., et al. (2022). Genistein effect on cognition in prodromal Alzheimer's disease patients. *The GENIAL clinical trial. Alzheimers Res Ther., 14*(1), 164.

Volkert, D., Kiesswetter, E., Cederholm, T., Donini, L. M., Eglseer, D., Norman, K., et al. (2019). Development of a model on determinants of malnutrition in aged persons: A MaNuEL project. *Gerontol Geriatr Med., 5*, 2333721419858438.

Wagle, A., Seong, S. H., Shrestha, S., Jung, H. A., & Choi, J. S. (2019). Korean thistle (Cirsium japonicum var. maackii (maxim.) Matsum.): A potential dietary supplement against diabetes and Alzheimer's disease. *Molecules, 24*(3), 649.

Waite, S. J., Maitland, S., Thomas, A., & Yarnall, A. J. (2021). Sarcopenia and frailty in individuals with dementia: A systematic review. *Archives of Gerontology and Geriatrics, 92*, 104268.

Wang, C., Fu, W., Cao, S., Jiang, H., Guo, Y., Xv, H., et al. (2021). Weight loss and the risk of dementia: A meta-analysis of cohort studies. *Current Alzheimer Research, 18*(2), 125–135.

Watson, R., & Deary, I. J. (1994). Measuring feeding difficulty in patients with dementia: Multivariate analysis of feeding problems, nursing intervention and indicators of feeding difficulty. *Journal of Advanced Nursing, 20*(2), 283–287.

White, H., Pieper, C., Schmader, K., & Fillenbaum, G. (1996). Weight change in Alzheimer's disease. *Journal of the American Geriatrics Society, 44*(3), 265–272.

World Health Organization. (2025, March 31). *Dementia [Internet]*. Retrieved August 26, 2025, from https://www.who.int/news-room/fact-sheets/detail/dementia

Chapter 9
Schizophrenia

Abstract

- Schizophrenia (SZ) is a chronic psychiatric disorder characterized by recurrent psychotic episodes, including positive symptoms (hallucinations, delusions), negative symptoms (anhedonia, flat affect, avolition), and cognitive impairments affecting attention, memory, and executive function.
- Approximately 24 million people worldwide are affected, with slightly higher prevalence in men and later age of diagnosis in women. Prognosis is generally worse in men.
- SZ arises from complex interactions of genetic (~80% heritability), environmental, biochemical, structural, and immunological factors. Over 130 genes affecting glutamatergic synapses and NMDA receptor function have been implicated. Prenatal exposures, nutritional deficiencies, vitamin D insufficiency, neuroinflammation, oxidative stress, and gut dysbiosis contribute to disease risk and progression.
- Nutritional management is essential as adjunct therapy to pharmacological treatment. Patients often exhibit poor dietary habits, low intake of folate, B6, B12, vitamin D, and polyunsaturated fatty acids, which exacerbate inflammation and neurotransmitter imbalances. Antipsychotic medications can cause metabolic side effects, increasing the need for dietary interventions.
- Recommended dietary approaches include Mediterranean, DASH, ketogenic, and, in some cases, gluten-free diets, emphasizing anti-inflammatory foods, adequate protein, omega-3 fatty acids, fiber, and hydration.
- Micronutrient supplementation (vitamins B, D, C, E, minerals such as zinc, selenium, and iron), antioxidants, melatonin, N-acetylcysteine, and polyphenols may improve cognitive, metabolic, and behavioral outcomes.
- Consideration of food–drug interactions is crucial, particularly with antipsychotics, SSRIs, and anxiolytics, to optimize therapeutic efficacy and minimize adverse effects.

M. H. Rouhani et al., *The Healing Plate*, SpringerBriefs in Modern Perspectives on Disability Research, https://doi.org/10.1007/978-981-95-8150-4_9

Keywords Schizophrenia (SZ) · Nutritional management · Antipsychotics · Micronutrients · Macronutrients · Food–drug interactions · Dietary patterns · Gut–brain axis · Oxidative stress · Mental health

9.1 Definition and Epidemiology

Schizophrenia (SZ) is a psychiatric condition characterized by persistent or recurrent episodes of psychosis, often leading to disruptions in social and occupational performance (Association AP, 2022). The clinical presentation of SZ commonly includes positive symptoms (such as hallucinations, delusions, and disorganized behavior), negative symptoms (anhedonia, lack of motivation, flat affect, and poverty of speech), and cognitive impairments (such as difficulties in attention, memory, and executive function) (Association AP, 2013).

Worldwide, nearly 24 million people live with SZ, representing around 0.32% of the population. In adults, this figure rises to 0.45% (Organization WH, 2022). SZ is diagnosed slightly more frequently in men than in women, with women typically receiving a diagnosis at a later age (Abel et al., 2010). Evidence suggests that the prognosis is worse in men (Grossman et al., 2008).

9.2 Etiology

SZ arises from complex interactions between genetic, environmental, biochemical, structural, and immunological factors, reflecting its heterogeneous nature (Altamura et al., 2013; Hany & StatPearls., 2025). Twin and family studies estimate that heritability accounts for approximately 80% of SZ risk (Marder & Cannon, 2019). Genome-wide association studies have identified over 130 genes related to neural differentiation, organization, and transmission, many of which affect glutamatergic synapses and N-methyl-D-aspartic acid (NMDA) receptor function (Coyle et al., 2020). Neuregulin 3, for instance, plays a key role in pyramidal neuron activation and proper glutamate transmission, and elevated levels are observed in patients with SZ.

Environmental factors also critically influence the onset and course of SZ. Prenatal exposures, including viral infections, ethanol, nutritional deficiencies, and perinatal complications, interact with genetic susceptibility to shape brain development (Davis et al., 2016; Maric & Svrakic, 2012).

Increasing evidence highlights the role of immunological and metabolic factors in SZ. Dysregulation of the gut microbiota, autoimmunity, neuroinflammation, oxidative stress, and epigenetic modifications, including DNA methylation and histone changes, have been implicated in disease pathogenesis. Moreover, lifestyle factors such as high-fat and high-sugar diets, as well as alcohol and opioid addictions, negatively affect adult neurogenesis and maintenance (Alam et al., 2017; Poulose et al., 2017; Severance et al., 2018). In addition, low vitamin D availability during brain development interacts with susceptibility genes to alter overall neurodevelopment. Vitamin D plays a crucial role in cell proliferation, differentiation, neuroprotection, neurotransmission, and neuroplasticity (S E-S., 2022).

9.3 Nutritional Management

Nutritional management is an essential part of SZ care, as medications alone cannot fully control symptoms, making dietary strategies necessary as complementary therapies (Arroll et al., 2014). In addition, nutritional quality is increasingly considered a risk factor for various psychiatric disorders, with individuals, including those with SZ, being more susceptible to poor dietary patterns (Tang et al., 2024). Therefore, initiating nutritional interventions early in the course of treatment may yield greater benefits for symptom management and long-term health, and this underscores the importance of involving a multidisciplinary team from the beginning of patient care (Teasdale et al., 2020).

9.3.1 Nutritional Challenges

Patients with SZ frequently exhibit unhealthy dietary habits and nutrient deficiencies, such as low levels of folate, vitamin B6, vitamin D, and polyunsaturated fatty acids (PUFAs) (Valipour et al., 2014; Cao et al., 2016; Tomioka et al., 2018; Teasdale et al., 2019; Ducrocq et al., 2020), which may exacerbate inflammation and neurochemical imbalances linked to symptomatology (Lopez-Garcia et al., 2004; Ryan et al., 2015). These dietary disturbances may arise from dysregulation of the brain's reward circuitry, including increased dopamine activity in the mesolimbic pathway and regions controlling cognition, contributing to obesity, food cravings, addictive behaviors, and other eating disorders (Onaolapo & Onaolapo, 2021). Moreover, insufficient intake or impaired absorption of folate and vitamin B12 can disrupt one-carbon metabolism, affecting nucleotide synthesis and elevating homocysteine levels, potentially increasing the risk of cardiovascular disease (Kale et al., 2010; Raghubeer & Matsha, 2021). The tryptophan/kynurenine metabolic pathway, crucial for amino acid metabolism, also appears abnormal in SZ, influenced by inflammation, stress, genetic factors, and brain-specific immune processes, highlighting the complex role of nutrition in this disorder (Yan et al., 2024). There is evidence suggesting a higher incidence of coeliac disease and non-coeliac gluten sensitivity in SZ, which may further complicate dietary management (Cascella et al., 2011; Okusaga et al., 2013). Alcohol consumption, prevalent among some patients, can additionally impair nutrient absorption and exacerbate existing deficiencies (Yan et al., 2024). Moreover, diet may influence SZ progression partly through the gut–brain axis, where dysbiosis can increase susceptibility to infection and inflammation, thereby accelerating disease development and aggravating symptom severity (Cha & Yang, 2020). In addition, antipsychotic medications often contribute to significant metabolic side effects including weight gain, dyslipidemia, and insulin resistance, further underscoring the importance of nutritional interventions (Libowitz & Nurmi, 2021).

9.3.2 General Dietary Recommendations

In general, it is recommended to include anti-inflammatory nutrients and foods as part of a balanced diet, as they may help reduce medication-related side effects, alleviate symptom severity, and lower risk factors associated with SZ (Rarinca et al., 2024). Adequate hydration and management of issues such as constipation or fecal impaction are also important considerations (S E-S., 2022). Therefore, treatment is generally recommended to be individualized, taking into account diagnosed nutritional deficiencies, physiological abnormalities, unique microbiome profiles, and inflammatory markers (Teasdale et al., 2020).

9.3.3 Dietary Patterns

Mediterranean and DASH Diet: In nutritional management of patients with SZ, adoption of healthy dietary patterns such as the Mediterranean and DASH diets is recommended to improve immune function, reduce metabolic risk, and lower cardiovascular comorbidities (Sorić et al., 2019).

Gluten-free Diet: Gluten-free diets may be considered to improve functioning or reduce symptom severity in SZ, although overall evidence is inconsistent (Onaolapo & Onaolapo, 2021).

Ketogenic Diet: Mechanistically, the ketogenic diet may modulate neurotransmitter balance, particularly the ratio of γ-aminobutyric acid (GABA) to glutamate, which can influence dopamine regulation (Steiniger & Kretschmer, 2003; Calderón et al., 2017). Additionally, it exhibits anti-inflammatory properties, with preclinical studies showing reduced plasma TNF-α and brain IL-1β levels (Dupuis et al., 2015). Although clinical evidence in SZ is limited, case studies have reported improvements in symptoms (Kraft & Westman, 2009).

9.3.4 Energy and Macronutrients Requirements

Caloric Intake: Individuals with SZ may exhibit altered energy intake, with a recent meta-analysis reporting an average additional consumption of +1695 kJ per day compared to healthy controls (Teasdale et al., 2019). This increased intake is often compounded by the effects of antipsychotic medications, which can lead to side effects such as heightened appetite and weight gain. These drugs interfere with energy balance both directly, by acting on hypothalamic and reward-related brain regions, and indirectly, by altering gut microbiota composition (Lu et al., 2015; Manu et al., 2015; Huang et al., 2020).

Protein: Adequate protein intake supports cognitive function, including executive function and memory, in SZ (Zhang et al., 2024). Balanced dietary interventions that include plant-based foods and high-quality, may help prevent SZ onset or delay symptom progression (Tang et al., 2024). A high-protein diet supports maintenance of muscle mass, reduces body fat, stabilizes blood glucose levels, decreases systemic inflammation, and enhances neural function (Leidy et al., 2015; Dickerson et al., 2020). Furthermore, emerging evidence suggests that supplementation with specific amino acids, including tryptophan and L-theanine, or glycine transporter type 1 (GlyT1) inhibitors can improve SZ symptoms, though optimal dosages may vary depending on the amino acid used (Arroll et al., 2014; Tang et al., 2024; Davidson et al., 2022).

Carbohydrate: Diets high in simple carbohydrates may elevate peripheral inflammatory markers, whereas fiber-rich foods and vegetables are associated with reduced inflammation (Firth et al., 2019).

Fat: Omega-3 PUFAs, primarily obtained from fatty fish, are essential for neurogenesis, neurotransmission, neuroinflammation, and overall brain development. Deficiency of these fatty acids has been observed in patients with SZ, contributing to altered membrane phospholipids, impaired neurotransmission, immune dysregulation, and reduced antioxidant defense (Hedelin et al., 2010; Lange, 2020). At the same time, reducing excess omega-6 fatty acids, common in industrial seed oils, is important to restore balance and support optimal neuronal function (Blasbalg et al., 2011).

9.3.5 Micronutrients Requirements and Supplementations

B vitamins: Particularly folate, vitamin B6, and vitamin B12 are essential for one-carbon metabolism, neurotransmitter synthesis, and homocysteine regulation (Kale et al., 2010; Calderón-Ospina & Nava-Mesa, 2020); low serum levels of these vitamins are not only commonly observed in patients with SZ but have also been linked to an increased risk of developing the disorder (Teasdale et al., 2020). Findings regarding supplementation with these vitamins in SZ remain contradictory (Brown & Roffman, 2014; Chen et al., 2024).

Vitamin D: An essential neurosteroid that regulates neurotransmitters and neurotrophic factors, thereby influencing brain plasticity (Garcion et al., 2002). Low vitamin D status is considered a risk factor for SZ, and a deficiency, which is highly prevalent among affected individuals, is linked to neurochemical and behavioral alterations (Ryan et al., 2015; Belbasis et al., 2018). However, findings on supplementation remain contradictory, with outcomes largely depending on dose and duration of administration (Brown & Roffman, 2014; Neriman et al., 2021).

Antioxidant vitamins: Deficiencies or low circulating levels of vitamins C, E, and beta-carotene contribute to increased oxidative stress (Brown & Roffman, 2014). Patients with SZ often present with elevated lipid peroxidation and altered antioxidant status, including changes in plasma and brain concentrations or in antioxidant enzyme activity (Steullet et al., 2017; An et al., 2018; Fraguas et al., 2019; Madireddy & Madireddy, 2020). Research indicates that antioxidant vitamins, particularly C and E, can protect cells from damage caused by inflammation and reactive oxygen species (Brown & Roffman, 2014). Vitamin C appeared beneficial across various doses, whereas outcomes for vitamin E were more variable, likely due to its pro-oxidant effects at high doses (Brown & Roffman, 2014).

Minerals: Deficiencies or excesses of essential trace elements, including calcium, zinc, selenium, copper, and manganese, have been reported in individuals with SZ, although the precise relationship between these elements and the disorder remains unclear (Tang et al., 2024; Onaolapo & Onaolapo, 2021; Rahman et al., 2009). In clinical research, administration of zinc sulfate (220 mg every 8 hours) was associated with improvement in SZ symptoms (Behrouzian et al., 2022), and selenium, alone or with probiotics, may improve Positive and Negative Syndrome Scale (PANSS) scores, memory, appetite, and some metabolic outcomes (Vaddadi et al., 2003; Jamilian & Ghaderi, 2021). Additionally, iron deficiency may contribute to cortical dopamine dysregulation and negative symptoms (Kim et al., 2018).

Melatonin (N-acetyl-5-methoxytryptamine): A naturally occurring compound that plays a key role in regulating the sleep–wake cycle (circadian rhythm) and acts as a potent antioxidant, both by directly scavenging free radicals and stimulating antioxidant enzymes. It also enhances intracellular glutathione (GSH) levels and stabilizes cellular membranes (Reiter et al., 2001). Nocturnal melatonin secretion has been found to be reduced in drug-free patients with SZ, and some antipsychotics, particularly olanzapine, further decrease melatonin levels, which may contribute to metabolic dysregulation and weight gain in treated patients (Arroll et al., 2014; Dodd et al., 2013). Supplementation with melatonin has been observed to improve sleep quality, increase morning freshness, enhance mood, and support daytime functioning in patients with SZ (Anderson & Maes, 2012).

Alpha-lipoic acid (ALA): A potent antioxidant capable of crossing the blood–brain barrier and performing functions similar to glutathione (Superti & Russo, 2024). In clinical studies, ALA supplementation has been associated with weight reduction, improved cholesterol levels, and increased energy, although its effects on core SZ symptoms remain limited (Foufelle & Ferré, 2005; Kim et al., 2008).

N-acetyl cysteine (NAC): Glutathione (GSH), a key antioxidant and free radical scavenger, is reduced in the brains of individuals with SZ (Yao et al., 2006; Gawryluk et al., 2011). NAC, a precursor of GSH, can effectively raise plasma glutathione levels. Studies have shown that NAC supplementation, at doses up to 2 g/day, can improve negative and general symptoms as well as overall functioning when used as an adjunct to antipsychotic therapy. Positive symptoms are generally less affected, but NAC may also support social functioning and overall well-being (Arroll et al., 2014).

Polyphenols: Patients may be encouraged to consume polyphenols, such as resveratrol, curcumin, blueberry polyphenols, and sulforaphane, to potentially support antioxidant defenses (S E-S., 2022).

9.4 Food–Drug Interactions

Currently, there is no cure for SZ and no medication that can directly reverse the course of the disease. However, pharmacological treatments can help manage its associated symptoms, including psychosis (such as hallucinations and delusions), depression, and anxiety. Table 9.1 provides a summary of the main drug classes used in SZ, their common examples, and relevant considerations for food–drug interactions (Library VH, n.d.; WebMD, n.d.; Kane & Correll, 2010; Abou-Setta et al., 2012; IA A, 2014; Remington et al., 2017; Mahan, 2020; Chokhawala, 2023; Sharbaf Shoar & Padhy, 2023; Singh, 2023; Bounds, 2024; Drugs.com, 2025a; Drugs.com, 2025b; Drugs.com, 2025c).

Table 9.1 Commonly prescribed medications for schizophrenia and their food–drug interactions

Drug	Trade name	Food–drug interactions
First-generation Antipsychotics		
Haloperidol	Haldol	**Side effects:** Dry mouth, constipation, and urinary retention **Avoid:** Alcohol
Chlorpromazine	Thorazine	Similar to Haloperidol
Second-generation Antipsychotics		
Clozapine	Clozaril	**Side effects:** Weight gain and the development of metabolic syndrome **Avoid:** Alcohol
Aripiprazole	Abilify	Similar to Clozapine
Antidepressants		
Sertraline (*SSRI*)	Zoloft	**Side effects:** Nausea, diarrhea, somnolence, tremor, fatigue **Avoid:** Tryptophan, alcohol, St John's wort, grapefruit juice, and herbal products that have antiplatelet effects
Citalopram (*SSRI*)	Celexa	**Side effects:** Drowsiness, insomnia, dizziness, headache, diaphoresis, nausea, vomiting, xerostomia, constipation, and diarrhea **Avoid:** Tryptophan, alcohol, St John's wort, and herbal products that have antiplatelet effects

(continued)

Table 9.1 (continued)

Drug	Trade name	Food–drug interactions
Fluoxetine (*SSRI*)	Prozac	**Side effects:** Anorexia, dry mouth **Avoid:** Tryptophan, alcohol, and herbal products that have antiplatelet effects
Anxiolytics		
Alprazolam	Xanax	**Side effects:** Respiratory depression, respiratory arrest, drowsiness, confusion, headache, syncope, nausea and vomiting, diarrhea, and tremors **Avoid:** Alcohol, caffeine, herbal, and natural products that cause CNS stimulation or sedation
Diazepam	Valium	Similar to Alprazolam
Lorazepam	Ativan	Similar to Alprazolam
Clonazepam	Restoril	Similar to Alprazolam

Acknowledgments The authors confirm that the content, analysis, and conclusions of this manuscript are their own work. AI-based tools were used solely to assist in improving the clarity and correctness of the English language.

References

Abel, K. M., Drake, R., & Goldstein, J. M. (2010). Sex differences in schizophrenia. *International Review of Psychiatry, 22*(5), 417–428.

Abou-Setta, A. M., Mousavi, S. S., & Spooner, C. (2012). *First-generation versus second-generation antipsychotics in adults: comparative effectiveness*. Comparative Effectiveness Reviews, No 63. Agency for Healthcare Research and Quality (US).

Alam, R., Abdolmaleky, H. M., & Zhou, J. R. (2017). Microbiome, inflammation, epigenetic alterations, and mental diseases. *American Journal of Medical Genetics. Part B, Neuropsychiatric Genetics, 174*(6), 651–660.

Altamura, A. C., Pozzoli, S., Fiorentini, A., & Dell'osso, B. (2013). Neurodevelopment and inflammatory patterns in schizophrenia in relation to pathophysiology. *Progress in Neuro-Psychopharmacology & Biological Psychiatry, 42*, 63–70.

An, H., Du, X., Huang, X., Qi, L., Jia, Q., Yin, G., et al. (2018). Obesity, altered oxidative stress, and clinical correlates in chronic schizophrenia patients. *Translational Psychiatry, 8*(1), 258.

Anderson, G., & Maes, M. (2012). Melatonin: an overlooked factor in schizophrenia and in the inhibition of anti-psychotic side effects. *Metabolic Brain Disease, 27*(2), 113–119.

Arroll, M. A., Wilder, L., & Neil, J. (2014). Nutritional interventions for the adjunctive treatment of schizophrenia: a brief review. *Nutrition Journal, 13*, 91.

Association AP. (2013). *Diagnostic and statistical manual of mental disorders* (5th ed.). American Psychiatric Association.

Association AP. (2022). *Diagnostic and statistical manual of mental disorders* (5th text revision ed.). American Psychiatric Association.

Behrouzian, F., Nazarinasab, M., Sadegh, A. M., Abdi, L., & Sabzevarizadeh, M. (2022). Effects of zinc sulfate on schizophrenia symptoms in patients undergoing atypical antipsychotic pharmacotherapy. *Journal of Family Medicine and Primary Care, 11*(12), 7795–7799.

Belbasis, L., Köhler, C. A., Stefanis, N., Stubbs, B., van Os, J., Vieta, E., et al. (2018). Risk factors and peripheral biomarkers for schizophrenia spectrum disorders: an umbrella review of meta-analyses. *Acta Psychiatrica Scandinavica, 137*(2), 88–97.

Blasbalg, T. L., Hibbeln, J. R., Ramsden, C. E., Majchrzak, S. F., & Rawlings, R. R. (2011). Changes in consumption of omega-3 and omega-6 fatty acids in the United States during the 20th century. *The American Journal of Clinical Nutrition, 93*(5), 950–962.

Bounds, C. G. P. P. (2024). *Benzodiazepines*. StatPearls [Internet]. Treasure Island (FL): StatPearls Publishing.

Brown, H. E., & Roffman, J. L. (2014). Vitamin supplementation in the treatment of schizophrenia. *CNS Drugs, 28*(7), 611–622.

Calderón, N., Betancourt, L., Hernández, L., & Rada, P. (2017). A ketogenic diet modifies glutamate, gamma-aminobutyric acid and agmatine levels in the hippocampus of rats: A microdialysis study. *Neuroscience Letters, 642*, 158–162.

Calderón-Ospina, C. A., & Nava-Mesa, M. O. (2020). B Vitamins in the nervous system: Current knowledge of the biochemical modes of action and synergies of thiamine, pyridoxine, and cobalamin. *CNS Neuroscience & Therapeutics, 26*(1), 5–13.

Cao, B., Wang, D. F., Xu, M. Y., Liu, Y. Q., Yan, L. L., Wang, J. Y., et al. (2016). Vitamin B12 and the risk of schizophrenia: A meta-analysis. *Schizophrenia Research, 172*(1–3), 216–217.

Cascella, N. G., Kryszak, D., Bhatti, B., Gregory, P., Kelly, D. L., Mc Evoy, J. P., et al. (2011). Prevalence of celiac disease and gluten sensitivity in the United States clinical antipsychotic trials of intervention effectiveness study population. *Schizophrenia Bulletin, 37*(1), 94–100.

Cha, H. Y., & Yang, S. J. (2020). Anti-Inflammatory Diets and Schizophrenia. *Clin Nutr Res., 9*(4), 241–257.

Chen, C. H., Chiu, C. C., Chiu, Y. H., Chang, C. H., Chang, Y. H., Huang, M. C., et al. (2024). Folate and vitamin B12 supplementation in patients with schizophrenia and low serum folate level: A 24-week randomized, double-blind, placebo-controlled study. *Journal of the Formosan Medical Association, 125*(1), 66–71.

Chokhawala, K. S. L. (2023). *Antipsychotic medications*. StatPearls [Internet]. Treasure Island (FL): StatPearls Publishing.

Coyle, J. T., Ruzicka, W. B., & Balu, D. T. (2020). Fifty Years of Research on Schizophrenia: The Ascendance of the Glutamatergic Synapse. *The American Journal of Psychiatry, 177*(12), 1119–1128.

Davidson, M., Rashidi, N., Nurgali, K., & Apostolopoulos, V. (2022). The Role of Tryptophan Metabolites in Neuropsychiatric Disorders. *International Journal of Molecular Sciences, 23*(17), 9968.

Davis, J., Eyre, H., Jacka, F. N., Dodd, S., Dean, O., McEwen, S., et al. (2016). A review of vulnerability and risks for schizophrenia: Beyond the two hit hypothesis. *Neuroscience and Biobehavioral Reviews, 65*, 185–194.

Dickerson, F., Gennusa, J. V., 3rd, Stallings, C., Origoni, A., Katsafanas, E., Sweeney, K., et al. (2020). Protein intake is associated with cognitive functioning in individuals with psychiatric disorders. *Psychiatry Research, 284*, 112700.

Dodd, S., Maes, M., Anderson, G., Dean, O. M., Moylan, S., & Berk, M. (2013). Putative neuroprotective agents in neuropsychiatric disorders. *Progress in Neuro-Psychopharmacology & Biological Psychiatry, 42*, 135–145.

Drugs.com. (2025a). *Aripiprazole: Food interactions: Drugs.com*. https://www.drugs.com/food-interactions/aripiprazole.html.

Drugs.com. (2025b). *Chlorpromazine: Food interactions: Drugs.com*. https://www.drugs.com/food-interactions/chlorpromazine.html.

Drugs.com. (2025c). *Clozapine: Food interactions: Drugs.com*. https://www.drugs.com/food-interactions/clozapine.html.

Ducrocq, F., Walle, R., Contini, A., Oummadi, A., Caraballo, B., van Der Veldt, S., et al. (2020). Causal link between n-3 polyunsaturated fatty acid deficiency and motivation deficits. *Cell Metabolism, 31*(4), 755–772. e7.

Dupuis, N., Curatolo, N., Benoist, J. F., & Auvin, S. (2015). Ketogenic diet exhibits anti-inflammatory properties. *Epilepsia, 56*(7), e95–e98.

Firth, J., Veronese, N., Cotter, J., Shivappa, N., Hebert, J. R., Ee, C., et al. (2019). What Is the Role of Dietary Inflammation in Severe Mental Illness? A Review of Observational and Experimental Findings. *Frontiers in Psychiatry, 10*, 350.

Foufelle, F., & Ferré, P. (2005). Role of adenosine monophosphate-activated protein kinase in the control of energy homeostasis. *Current Opinion in Clinical Nutrition and Metabolic Care, 8*(4), 355–360.

Fraguas, D., Díaz-Caneja, C. M., Ayora, M., Hernández-Álvarez, F., Rodríguez-Quiroga, A., Recio, S., et al. (2019). Oxidative Stress and Inflammation in First-Episode Psychosis: A Systematic Review and Meta-analysis. *Schizophrenia Bulletin, 45*(4), 742–751.

Garcion, E., Wion-Barbot, N., Montero-Menei, C. N., Berger, F., & Wion, D. (2002). New clues about vitamin D functions in the nervous system. *Trends in Endocrinology and Metabolism, 13*(3), 100–105.

Gawryluk, J. W., Wang, J. F., Andreazza, A. C., Shao, L., & Young, L. T. (2011). Decreased levels of glutathione, the major brain antioxidant, in post-mortem prefrontal cortex from patients with psychiatric disorders. *The International Journal of Neuropsychopharmacology, 14*(1), 123–130.

Grossman, L. S., Harrow, M., Rosen, C., Faull, R., & Strauss, G. P. (2008). Sex differences in schizophrenia and other psychotic disorders: a 20-year longitudinal study of psychosis and recovery. *Comprehensive Psychiatry, 49*(6), 523–529.

Hany, M., & Rizvi, A. (2025). *Schizophrenia*. StatPearls. Treasure Island (FL): StatPearls Publishing Copyright © 2025, StatPearls Publishing LLC.

Hedelin, M., Löf, M., Olsson, M., Lewander, T., Nilsson, B., Hultman, C. M., et al. (2010). Dietary intake of fish, omega-3, omega-6 polyunsaturated fatty acids and vitamin D and the prevalence of psychotic-like symptoms in a cohort of 33,000 women from the general population. *BMC Psychiatry, 10*, 38.

Huang, J., Hei, G. R., Yang, Y., Liu, C. C., Xiao, J. M., Long, Y. J., et al. (2020). Increased Appetite Plays a Key Role in Olanzapine-Induced Weight Gain in First-Episode Schizophrenia Patients. *Frontiers in Pharmacology, 11*, 739.

IA A. (2014). *Food-drug interactions and their impact on the pharmacotherapy.* University of Veterinary and Pharmaceutical Sciences Brno, Faculty of Pharmacy, Department of Human Pharmacology and Toxicology.

Jamilian, H., & Ghaderi, A. (2021). The Effects of Probiotic and Selenium Co-supplementation on Clinical and Metabolic Scales in Chronic Schizophrenia: a Randomized, Double-blind. *Placebo-Controlled Trial. Biol Trace Elem Res., 199*(12), 4430–4438.

Kale, A., Naphade, N., Sapkale, S., Kamaraju, M., Pillai, A., Joshi, S., et al. (2010). Reduced folic acid, vitamin B12 and docosahexaenoic acid and increased homocysteine and cortisol in never-medicated schizophrenia patients: implications for altered one-carbon metabolism. *Psychiatry Research, 175*(1–2), 47–53.

Kane, J. M., & Correll, C. U. (2010). Pharmacologic treatment of schizophrenia. *Dialogues in Clinical Neuroscience, 12*(3), 345–357.

Kim, E., Park, D. W., Choi, S. H., Kim, J. J., & Cho, H. S. (2008). A preliminary investigation of alpha-lipoic acid treatment of antipsychotic drug-induced weight gain in patients with schizophrenia. *Journal of Clinical Psychopharmacology, 28*(2), 138–146.

Kim, S. W., Stewart, R., Park, W. Y., Jhon, M., Lee, J. Y., Kim, S. Y., et al. (2018). Latent Iron Deficiency as a Marker of Negative Symptoms in Patients with First-Episode Schizophrenia Spectrum Disorder. *Nutrients, 10*(11), 1707.

Kraft, B. D., & Westman, E. C. (2009). Schizophrenia, gluten, and low-carbohydrate, ketogenic diets: a case report and review of the literature. *Nutrition & Metabolism (London), 6*, 10.

Lange, K. W. (2020). Omega-3 fatty acids and mental health. *Global Health Journal., 4*(1), 18–30.

Leidy, H. J., Clifton, P. M., Astrup, A., Wycherley, T. P., Westerterp-Plantenga, M. S., Luscombe-Marsh, N. D., et al. (2015). The role of protein in weight loss and maintenance. *The American Journal of Clinical Nutrition, 101*(6), 1320s–1329s.

Libowitz, M. R., & Nurmi, E. L. (2021). The Burden of Antipsychotic-Induced Weight Gain and Metabolic Syndrome in Children. *Frontiers in Psychiatry, 12*, 623681.

Library VH. (n.d.). *Encyclopedia—Veterans health library.* https://www.veteranshealthlibrary.va.gov/Encyclopedia/142,AA47582_VA

Lopez-Garcia, E., Schulze, M. B., Fung, T. T., Meigs, J. B., Rifai, N., Manson, J. E., et al. (2004). Major dietary patterns are related to plasma concentrations of markers of inflammation and endothelial dysfunction. *The American Journal of Clinical Nutrition, 80*(4), 1029–1035.

Lu, M. L., Wang, T. N., Lin, T. Y., Shao, W. C., Chang, S. H., Chou, J. Y., et al. (2015). Differential effects of olanzapine and clozapine on plasma levels of adipocytokines and total ghrelin. *Progress in Neuro-Psychopharmacology & Biological Psychiatry, 58*, 47–50.

Madireddy, S., & Madireddy, S. (2020). Regulation of Reactive Oxygen Species-Mediated Damage in the Pathogenesis of Schizophrenia. *Brain Sciences, 10*(10), 742.

Mahan, L. K. R. J. (2020). *Krause's food & the nutrition care process* (15th ed.). Elsevier.

Manu, P., Dima, L., Shulman, M., Vancampfort, D., De Hert, M., & Correll, C. U. (2015). Weight gain and obesity in schizophrenia: epidemiology, pathobiology, and management. *Acta Psychiatrica Scandinavica, 132*(2), 97–108.

Marder, S. R., & Cannon, T. D. (2019). Schizophrenia. *The New England Journal of Medicine, 381*(18), 1753–1761.

Maric, N. P., & Svrakic, D. M. (2012). Why schizophrenia genetics needs epigenetics: a review. *Psychiatria Danubina, 24*(1), 2–18.

Neriman, A., Hakan, Y., & Ozge, U. (2021). The psychotropic effect of vitamin D supplementation on schizophrenia symptoms. *BMC Psychiatry, 21*(1), 309.

Okusaga, O., Yolken, R. H., Langenberg, P., Sleemi, A., Kelly, D. L., Vaswani, D., et al. (2013). Elevated gliadin antibody levels in individuals with schizophrenia. *The World Journal of Biological Psychiatry, 14*(7), 509–515.

Onaolapo, O. J., & Onaolapo, A. Y. (2021). Nutrition, nutritional deficiencies, and schizophrenia: An association worthy of constant reassessment. *World Journal of Clinical Cases, 9*(28), 8295–8311.

Organization WH. (2022). *Schizophrenia Geneva.* WHO. https://www.who.int/news-room/fact-sheets/detail/schizophrenia?utm_source=chatgpt.com

Poulose, S. M., Miller, M. G., Scott, T., & Shukitt-Hale, B. (2017). Nutritional Factors Affecting Adult Neurogenesis and Cognitive Function. *Advances in Nutrition, 8*(6), 804–811.

Raghubeer, S., & Matsha, T. E. (2021). Methylenetetrahydrofolate (MTHFR), the One-Carbon Cycle, and Cardiovascular Risks. *Nutrients, 13*(12), 4562.

Rahman, A., Azad, M. A., Hossain, I., Qusar, M. M., Bari, W., Begum, F., et al. (2009). Zinc, manganese, calcium, copper, and cadmium level in scalp hair samples of schizophrenic patients. *Biological Trace Element Research, 127*(2), 102–108.

Rarinca, V., Vasile, A., Visternicu, M., Burlui, V., Halitchi, G., Ciobica, A., et al. (2024). Relevance of diet in schizophrenia: a review focusing on prenatal nutritional deficiency, obesity, oxidative stress and inflammation. *Frontiers in Nutrition, 11*, 1497569.

Reiter, R. J., Acuña-Castroviejo, D., Tan, D. X., & Burkhardt, S. (2001). Free radical-mediated molecular damage. Mechanisms for the protective actions of melatonin in the central nervous system. *Annals of the New York Academy of Sciences, 939*, 200–215.

Remington, G., Addington, D., Honer, W., Ismail, Z., Raedler, T., & Teehan, M. (2017). Guidelines for the pharmacotherapy of schizophrenia in adults. *The Canadian Journal of Psychiatry., 62*(9), 604–616.

Ryan, J. W., Anderson, P. H., & Morris, H. A. (2015). Pleiotropic Activities of Vitamin D Receptors - Adequate Activation for Multiple Health Outcomes. *Clinical Biochemist Reviews, 36*(2), 53–61.

S E-S. (2022). *Nutrition & diagnosis-related care* (9th ed.). Academy of Nutrition and Dietetics.

Severance, E. G., Dickerson, F. B., & Yolken, R. H. (2018). Autoimmune phenotypes in schizophrenia reveal novel treatment targets. *Pharmacology & Therapeutics, 189*, 184–198.

Sharbaf Shoar, N. F. K., & Padhy, R. K. (2023). *Citalopram*. StatPearls [Internet]. Treasure Island (FL): StatPearls Publishing.

Singh, H. K. S. A. (2023). *Sertraline*. StatPearls [Internet]. Treasure Island (FL): StatPearls Publishing.

Sorić, T., Mavar, M., & Rumbak, I. (2019). The Effects of the Dietary Approaches to Stop Hypertension (DASH) Diet on Metabolic Syndrome in Hospitalized Schizophrenic Patients: A Randomized Controlled Trial. *Nutrients, 11*(12), 2950.

Steiniger, B., & Kretschmer, B. D. (2003). Glutamate and GABA modulate dopamine in the pedunculopontine tegmental nucleus. *Experimental Brain Research, 149*(4), 422–430.

Steullet, P., Cabungcal, J. H., Coyle, J., Didriksen, M., Gill, K., Grace, A. A., et al. (2017). Oxidative stress-driven parvalbumin interneuron impairment as a common mechanism in models of schizophrenia. *Molecular Psychiatry, 22*(7), 936–943.

Superti, F., & Russo, R. (2024). Alpha-Lipoic Acid: Biological Mechanisms and Health Benefits. *Antioxidants (Basel)., 13*(10), 1228.

Tang, M., Zhao, T., Liu, T., Dang, R., Cai, H., & Wang, Y. (2024). Nutrition and schizophrenia: associations worthy of continued revaluation. *Nutritional Neuroscience, 27*(6), 528–546.

Teasdale, S., Mörkl, S., & Müller-Stierlin, A. S. (2020). Nutritional psychiatry in the treatment of psychotic disorders: Current hypotheses and research challenges. *Brain Behav Immun Health., 5*, 100070.

Teasdale, S. B., Ward, P. B., Samaras, K., Firth, J., Stubbs, B., Tripodi, E., et al. (2019). Dietary intake of people with severe mental illness: systematic review and meta-analysis. *The British Journal of Psychiatry, 214*(5), 251–259.

Tomioka, Y., Numata, S., Kinoshita, M., Umehara, H., Watanabe, S. Y., Nakataki, M., et al. (2018). Decreased serum pyridoxal levels in schizophrenia: meta-analysis and Mendelian randomization analysis. *Journal of Psychiatry & Neuroscience, 43*(3), 194–200.

Vaddadi, K. S., Soosai, E., & Vaddadi, G. (2003). Low blood selenium concentrations in schizophrenic patients on clozapine. *British Journal of Clinical Pharmacology, 55*(3), 307–309.

Valipour, G., Saneei, P., & Esmaillzadeh, A. (2014). Serum vitamin D levels in relation to schizophrenia: a systematic review and meta-analysis of observational studies. *The Journal of Clinical Endocrinology and Metabolism, 99*(10), 3863–3872.

WebMD. (n.d.). *Medicines to treat schizophrenia: WebMD*. https://www.webmd.com/schizophrenia/medicines-to-treat-schizophrenia

Yan, Y., Zhou, D., & Chen, J. (2024). Navigating Nutritional Inequality in Schizophrenia: A Comprehensive Exploration of Diet, Genetics, and Holistic Management Across the Life Cycle. *Nutrients, 16*(21), 3738.

Yao, J. K., Leonard, S., & Reddy, R. (2006). Altered glutathione redox state in schizophrenia. *Disease Markers, 22*(1–2), 83–93.

Zhang, R., Zhang, B., Shen, C., Sahakian, B. J., Li, Z., Zhang, W., et al. (2024). Associations of dietary patterns with brain health from behavioral, neuroimaging, biochemical and genetic analyses. *Nature Mental Health, 2*(5), 535–552.

Chapter 10
Parkinson's Disease

Abstract

- Progressive motor, cognitive, and non-motor impairments in Parkinson's disease cause severe disability, dependence, and rising global prevalence.
- Multifactorial etiology includes genetics, environmental toxins, oxidative stress, mitochondrial dysfunction, neurotransmitter imbalance, and age-related dopaminergic neuron loss.
- Nutritional challenges involve anorexia, dysgeusia, dysphagia, constipation, dehydration, altered energy needs, and weight fluctuations.
- High-quality diets (Mediterranean, MIND, plant- and fish-rich) provide antioxidants, anti-inflammatory compounds, and neuroprotective benefits.
- Protein intake should be timed to optimize levodopa absorption: lower during the day, higher in the evening; adjust total intake based on weight and metabolism.
- Targeted nutrients: vitamin D, Folate, B12, antioxidants, and polyphenols support cognitive and motor function; high-dose B6 (>15 mg/day) should be avoided.
- Excess manganese, iron, or cysteine may worsen neurodegeneration; certain botanicals (Mucuna pruriens, Goji Berry, Ginkgo) show potential but require further research.
- Practical care: texture-modified meals, small frequent portions, hydration, constipation and xerostomia management, assisted feeding when needed, regular weight/BMI monitoring, and meals during optimal motor periods.
- Food–drug interactions are critical: levodopa, MAO-B inhibitors, entacapone, and other medications may require dietary adjustments to prevent absorption issues or adverse effects.
- Physical activity complements nutritional care, supporting overall function, mobility, and quality of life.

Keywords Parkinson disease · Neurodevelopmental disorders · Nutrition · Dietary patterns · Gastrointestinal disorders · Micronutrients · Food–drug interactions

M. H. Rouhani et al., *The Healing Plate*, SpringerBriefs in Modern Perspectives on Disability Research, https://doi.org/10.1007/978-981-95-8150-4_10

10.1 Definition and Epidemiology

Parkinson disease (PD) is a prevalent neurodegenerative and disabling disorder, widely recognized as a major cause of long-term disability worldwide. It imposes a significant disability burden and poses an escalating global public health challenge, marked by its triad of motor impairments, non-motor complications, and progressive cognitive decline (Morris et al., 2024). As a disability disorder, PD severely compromises mobility, independence, and quality of life, rendering patients increasingly dependent on caregivers and healthcare systems. The World Health Organization predicts that by 2040, neurodegenerative diseases, such as PD and Alzheimer's, will surpass cancer to become the second leading cause of death globally, marking a seismic shift in global health priorities (Su et al., 2025). Males are affected slightly more often than females. PD emerges as the fastest-growing neurological threat, with global case numbers projected to rise by 112% between 2021 and 2050, reaching 25.2 million, while age-standardized prevalence escalates to 216 per 100,000, cementing its status as a defining public health crisis of the twenty-first century (Su et al., 2025).

10.2 Etiology

The etiology of PD is multifactorial and not yet fully elucidated, but it is believed to arise from a complex interplay between genetic predisposition and environmental influences (Aquilani et al., 2008). Key contributing factors include genetic mutations, exposure to environmental toxins, prion-related protein misfolding, oxidative stress, and mitochondrial dysfunction, all of which can disrupt neuronal homeostasis. Additional mechanisms involve an imbalance of neurotransmitters leading to excitotoxicity, impaired neuroinflammatory regulation within specific brain regions, defective dopamine signaling, and an accelerated rate of neuronal apoptosis. Age-related degeneration of dopaminergic neurons further exacerbates disease progression. While twin and family studies highlight a stronger genetic component in early onset of PD, more than 16 mutations across multiple chromosomes have been identified, yet only 10–15% of cases are classified as familial (Aquilani et al., 2010). Genetic testing, however, is not part of routine clinical practice and remains primarily confined to research contexts.

10.3 Nutritional Management

10.3.1 Nutritional Challenges

PD profoundly elevates the risk of both malnutrition and dynamic weight changes, driven by a complex pathophysiological interplay. Core non-motor features such as anosmia, hypogeusia, and constipation directly suppress appetite and reduce nutritional intake, while heightened metabolic demands and motor complications like dyskinesias can create a chronic energy deficit, initially leading to weight loss that primarily involves fat mass (Mischley, 2017; Barichella et al., 2009; Cereda et al., 2012). This vulnerability is severely compounded by progressive motor impairments; resting tremors limit self-feeding, and dysphagia further restricts safe dietary intake and compromises hydration (Takizawa et al., 2016; Rodrigues et al., 2011). This necessitates proactive screening as it leads to reduced intake, dehydration, and aspiration pneumonia, the leading cause of PD mortality (Lethbridge et al., 2013). Conversely, therapeutic interventions, particularly deep brain stimulation, can paradoxically induce significant weight gain in advanced stages. This gain is largely attributed to reduced energy expenditure from controlled motor symptoms and changes in eating behavior, but it manifests primarily as abdominal fat, increasing the risk of metabolic syndrome (Aiello et al., 2015; Fasano et al., 2015; Rieu et al., 2011; Rimmelzwaan et al., 2016). Therefore, nutritional management must be meticulous and individualized, necessitating regular weight monitoring and annual nutritional assessments to effectively mitigate these dual and opposing risks.

10.3.2 General Dietary Recommendations

Evidence from large perspective cohorts and meta-analyses indicates that higher overall diet quality is associated with a reduced risk of PD and may delay its onset, while proinflammatory dietary patterns are linked to a higher risk of prodromal PD. Adherence to healthy patterns, particularly the Mediterranean diet, the MIND diet, and other prudent plant-based and fish-rich diets with limited processed and Western-type foods, consistently demonstrates inverse associations with both PD incidence and disease progression. Key components such as fruits, vegetables, green tea (Camellia sinensis), coffee, turmeric, nuts, and vegetable or olive oils provide antioxidant and anti-inflammatory benefits, and moderate caffeine intake has been associated with a 17% slower progression in early stage PD (Molsberry et al., 2020; Zhang et al., 2022; Metcalfe-Roach et al., 2021; Agarwal et al., 2018; Hosking et al., 2019).

10.3.3 Dietary Protein Intake

In advanced PD with motor fluctuations, careful protein management is critical, as excess intake can impair levodopa absorption. Daily protein should generally target 0.5 g/kg, increasing to 1–1.5 g/kg if unintentional weight loss occurs, while diets above 2 g/kg may reduce drug efficacy. A protein redistribution strategy, low-protein breakfast and lunch with higher protein in the evening, or a 7:1 carbohydrate-to-protein ratio is recommended to optimize levodopa response and may also help mitigate dyskinesia.

10.3.4 Targeted Nutrients and Supplements

Vitamin D: PD patients frequently present with low serum vitamin D levels (Barichella et al., 2017) and insufficient dietary intake, associated with increased disease risk, faster progression, and reduced bone mineral density, which raises fracture risk (Rimmelzwaan et al., 2016; Shen & Ji, 2015; van den Bos et al., 2013).

Vitamin B12 and Folate: Levodopa therapy elevates homocysteine (Hu et al., 2013), which may impair bone mineral density (Lee et al., 2010) and contribute to neuropathic complications (Bellomo et al., 2005; Wu et al., 2021). PD patients often exhibit reduced folate and B12 levels (Zoccolella et al., 2005; Triantafyllou et al., 2007). Supplementation with these vitamins is recommended to lower homocysteine levels (Hu et al., 2013; Lamberti et al., 2005; Postuma et al., 2006), and prevent related complications.

Pyridoxine (Vitamin B6): High-dose pyridoxine (>15 mg/day) accelerates peripheral conversion of L-dopa to dopamine, reducing its availability in the brain. Supplementation above 15 mg/day is not recommended.

Antioxidant-rich and Neuroprotective Nutrients: Nutrients such as glutathione, curcumin, omega-3 fatty acids, vitamins E, resveratrol, caffeine, and quercetin may modulate oxidative stress, inflammation, and apoptosis, though current evidence is inconclusive (Amro et al., 2018). Polyphenols like resveratrol (grapes, red wine), curcumin (turmeric), and epigallocatechin (green tea) may enhance neurotrophic factors and act synergistically with pharmacological treatments (Sun et al., 2008).

10.3.5 Key Botanicals and Phytochemicals with Neuroprotective Potential

Several studies have highlighted the potential role of medicinal plants in managing PD. However, their application necessitates further research to substantiate their beneficial effects. Certain plants that may offer potential benefits for PD include Mucuna pruriens (Velvet Bean), Lycium barbarum (Goji Berry), Peganum harmala (Syrian Rue), Carthamus tinctorius (Safflower), Baicalein (Scutellaria baicalensis), Pueraria lobata (Kudzu), Tianma Gouteng Yin, Chunghyuldan, and Ginkgo biloba (van den Bos et al., 2013). It is crucial to reiterate that the use of these plants is not yet established as a component of standard treatment for PD patients, and more extensive studies are required in this area. Consequently, their use for PD management outside of formal clinical trials is not recommended.

10.3.6 Nutrients with Unfavorable Accumulation

Manganese (Mn): Excess Mn from occupational exposure or parenteral nutrition accumulates in the basal ganglia, causing Parkinson-like symptoms (tremor, rigidity, gait disturbance). Even chronic low doses (~0.1 mg/day) can lead to deposition (Sandström et al., 1987). Manganese should be carefully monitored to avoid excesses above dietary reference intake levels.

Cysteine: Elevated plasma levels are linked with PD and Alzheimer's diseases (Heafield et al., 1990).

Iron: Emerging evidence indicates that excessive iron deposition may increase vulnerability to neurodegenerative conditions, including PD, Alzheimer's disease, and age-related macular degeneration (Belaidi & Bush, 2016; Fleming & Ponka, 2012).

10.3.7 Practical Feeding and Care Guidelines

The key nutritional concerns that must be evaluated in patients with PD are outlined in the Fig. 10.1. For each patient, the degree and severity of these issues should be assessed through personalized interventions, and a tailored nutritional plan should be developed to manage them. The following practical approaches provide specific strategies for managing the most common nutritional challenges in patients with PD.

- **Constipation Management**

  Promote high-fiber intake, gradually increasing it in patients with gastroparesis, along with hydration and regular exercise; use bran, prune juice, laxatives, or pre/probiotics as needed, and monitor weight to prevent malnutrition.

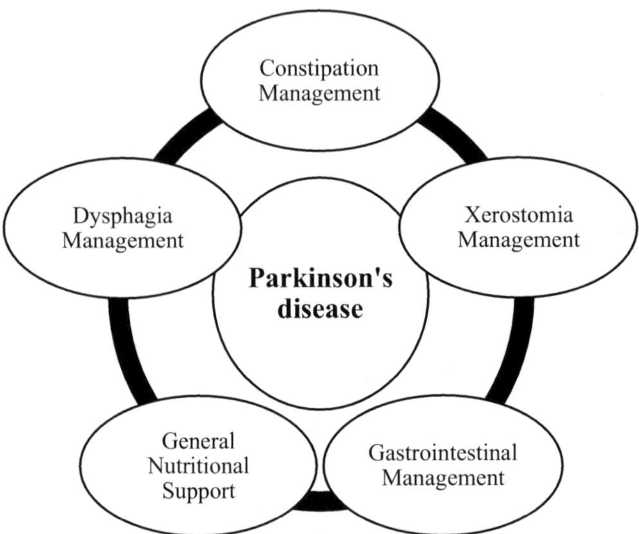

Fig. 10.1 Key nutritional concerns in PD

- **Dysphagia (Swallowing Difficulties) Management**
  Adapt food texture, provide small frequent meals, and offer feeding support. Screen regularly to prevent aspiration, consider enteral nutrition in the case of severe gastroparesis or inadequate intakes, and optimize meal timing and protein distribution to support motor function.
- **Xerostomia (Dry Mouth) Management**
  Stimulate saliva with tart foods, maintain hydration using small sips or ice chips, and consider a cool-mist humidifier at night. Use straws, rinse with mild saline, and add sauces or gravies to ease swallowing. Avoid caffeine, alcohol, and tobacco.
- **Management of Other Gastrointestinal Disorders**
  Focus on improving gastric emptying and reducing upper GI discomfort by encouraging small, frequent, low-fat, and low-fiber meals. Minimize gastric irritants such as spices, coffee, and alcohol. Consider enteral feeding (duodenal or PEG) if gastroparesis persists or oral intake is insufficient. Regularly monitor weight and BMI to prevent malnutrition.
- **General Nutritional Support and Monitoring**
  Comprehensive nutritional support for Parkinson's patients is essential and includes regular weight and BMI monitoring to proactively prevent malnutrition. To optimize intake, meals should be scheduled during "on" periods of optimal motor function and energy, with assistance provided during eating to extend mealtimes and significantly improve caloric and protein consumption for those with fatigue or impairment. For patients experiencing severe motor fluctuations, a dietary strategy of reduced daytime protein intake, with unrestricted intake in the evening, can be considered. Alongside these nutritional measures, patients are strongly advised to

engage in at least 150 min of moderate-intensity aerobic exercise weekly to support overall management of the condition (Corcos et al., 2024).

10.4 Food–Drug Interactions

Optimizing PD therapy is crucial to overcome limitations such as insufficient symptom control, poor adherence in advanced stages, and variable individual responses. Aligning medication intake with meals and managing food–drug interactions can enhance treatment efficacy. Table 10.1 summarizes major PD drug classes, representative examples, and key considerations for potential food–drug interactions, offering a practical guide to integrate nutritional strategies into comprehensive PD management (Agnieszka et al., 2022).

Table 10.1 Commonly prescribed medications for parkinson disease and their food–drug interactions

Drug	Trade name	Food–drug interactions
Dopamine agonists		
Apomorphine	Apokyn	**Side effects:** Nausea, vomiting, weight gain, lack of appetite **Avoid:** Alcohol
Pramipexole	Mirapex	**Side effects:** Nausea, constipation **Avoid:** Alcohol
Ropinirole	Requip	**Side effects:** Nausea, abdominal pain, constipation, diarrhea, dyspepsia **Avoid:** Alcohol
Levodopa and carbidopa		
Carbidopa/levodopa	Sinemet	**Side effects:** Hypokalemia, anorexia, nausea, and vomiting, associated with GI irritation (bleeding and/or ulceration) **Avoid:** Alcohol, high protein diets, and avoid large fluctuations in daily protein, high-fiber diets, vitamin B6, and mineral supplements (Fe)
Foscarbidopa/foslevodopa	Vyalev	**Side effects:** Constipation, diarrhea, dry mouth, dysgeusia, dyspepsia, dysphagia, flatulence, nausea, and vomiting **Avoid:** Alcohol
Monoamine oxidase-B inhibitors) MAO-B (		
Selegiline	Eldepryl	**Side effects:** Xerostomia, nausea and vomiting, loss of appetite **Avoid:** Alcohol, caffein, foods containing high amounts of tyramine such as air dried meats, aged or fermented meats, sausage or salami, pickled herring, any spoiled or improperly stored beef, poultry, fish, or liver, red wine, beer from a tap, unpasteurized beer, aged cheeses including blue, brick, brie, cheddar, parmesan, Romano, and Swiss, sauerkraut, over-the-counter supplements or cough and cold medicines that contain tyramine, soy beans, soy sauce, tofu, miso soup, bean curd, fava beans, yeast extracts (such as marmite)

(continued)

Table 10.1 (continued)

Drug	Trade name	Food–drug interactions
Rasagiline	Azilect	**Side effects:** Abdominal pain, anorexia, constipation, diarrhea, dyspepsia, dysphagia, nausea, and vomiting **Avoid** alcohol, caffeine, foods containing high amounts of tyramine such as air dried meats, aged or fermented meats, sausage or salami, pickled herring, any spoiled or improperly stored beef, poultry, fish, or liver, red wine, beer from a tap, unpasteurized beer, aged cheeses including blue, brick, brie, cheddar, parmesan, Romano, and Swiss, sauerkraut, over-the-counter supplements or cough and cold medicines that contain tyramine, soy beans, soy sauce, tofu, miso soup, bean curd, fava beans, yeast extracts (such as marmite)
Safinamide	Xadago	**Side effects:** Nausea and vomiting, dyspepsia **Avoid** alcohol, foods containing high amounts of tyramine such as air dried meats, aged or fermented meats, sausage or salami, pickled herring, any spoiled or improperly stored beef, poultry, fish, or liver, red wine, beer from a tap, unpasteurized beer, aged cheeses including blue, brick, brie, cheddar, parmesan, Romano, and Swiss, sauerkraut, over-the-counter supplements or cough and cold medicines that contain tyramine, soy beans, soy sauce, tofu, miso soup, bean curd, fava beans, yeast extracts (such as marmite)
Catechol-O-methyltransferase inhibitors (COMT)		
Entacapone	Comtan	**Side effects:** Constipation, diarrhea, dizziness, nausea, abdominal pain **Avoid** alcohol, iron
Opicapone	Ongentys	**Side effects:** Constipation, weight loss, xerostomia **Avoid:** Alcohol
Tolcapone	Tasmar	**Side effects:** Diarrhea, nausea, vomiting, and loss of appetite **Avoid:** Alcohol
Adamantanes		
Amantadine	Symmetrel	**Side effects:** Nausea, constipation, and weight loss **Avoid:** Alcohol
Anticholinergics		
Benztropine	Cogentin	**Side effects:** Loss of appetite and weight, decreased GI motility (constipation) **Avoid:** Alcohol
Trihexyphenidyl	Artane	**Side effects:** Decreased GI motility (constipation) **Avoid:** Alcohol
Adenosine A2A antagonists		
Istradefylline	Nourianz	**Side effects:** Constipation, loss of appetite, xerostomia, nausea **Avoid**: St. John's wort, grapefruit juice
Others		
Methylphenidate	Ritalin	**Side effects:** Anorexia and weight loss **Avoid**: Caffeine, alcohol
Polyethylene glycol	MiraLAX	**Side effects:** Nausea or vomiting, stomach cramps **Avoid:** Alcohol

(continued)

Table 10.1 (continued)

Drug	Trade name	Food–drug interactions
Modafinil	Provigil	**Side effects:** Nausea **Avoid:** Alcohol
Diazepam	Valium	**Side effects:** Anorexia **Avoid:** Alcohol, grapefruit or grapefruit juice, and caffeine
Orphenadrine	Norflex	**Side effects:** Xerostomia, nausea and vomiting, constipation **Avoid:** Alcohol
Carbamazepine	Tegretol	**Side effects:** Weight gain and causes nutrient depletions (folic acid, biotin, and vitamin D) **Avoid:** St John's wort, grapefruit juice, pomegranate juice, and alcohol
Amitriptyline (TCA)	Elavil	**Side effects:** Urinary retention, constipation **Avoid:** Alcohol

Acknowledgments The authors confirm that the content, analysis, and conclusions of this manuscript are their own work. AI-based tools were used solely to assist in improving the clarity and correctness of the English language.

References

Agarwal, P., Wang, Y., Buchman, A. S., Holland, T. M., Bennett, D. A., & Morris, M. C. (2018). MIND diet associated with reduced incidence and delayed progression of ParkinsonismA in old age. *The Journal of Nutrition, Health & Aging, 22*(10), 1211–1215.

Agnieszka, W., Paweł, P., & Małgorzata, K. (2022). How to optimize the effectiveness and safety of Parkinson's disease therapy?—A systematic review of drugs interactions with food and dietary supplements. *Current Neuropharmacology, 20*(7), 1427–1447.

Aiello, M., Eleopra, R., & Rumiati, R. I. (2015). Body weight and food intake in Parkinson's disease. A review of the association to non-motor symptoms. *Appetite, 84*, 204–211.

Amro, M. S., Teoh, S. L., Norzana, A. G., & Srijit, D. (2018). The potential role of herbal products in the treatment of Parkinson's disease. *La Clinica Terapeutica, 169*(1), e23–e33.

Aquilani, R., Scocchi, M., Boschi, F., Viglio, S., Iadarola, P., Pastoris, O., et al. (2008). Effect of calorie-protein supplementation on the cognitive recovery of patients with subacute stroke. *Nutritional Neuroscience, 11*(5), 235–240.

Aquilani, R., Scocchi, M., Iadarola, P., Viglio, S., Pasini, E., Condello, S., et al. (2010). Spontaneous neurocognitive retrieval of patients with sub-acute ischemic stroke is associated with dietary protein intake. *Nutritional Neuroscience, 13*(3), 129–134.

Barichella, M., Cereda, E., Cassani, E., Pinelli, G., Iorio, L., Ferri, V., et al. (2017). Dietary habits and neurological features of Parkinson's disease patients: Implications for practice. *Clinical Nutrition, 36*(4), 1054–1061.

Barichella, M., Cereda, E., & Pezzoli, G. (2009). Major nutritional issues in the management of Parkinson's disease. *Movement Disorders, 24*(13), 1881–1892.

Belaidi, A. A., & Bush, A. I. (2016). Iron neurochemistry in Alzheimer's disease and Parkinson's disease: Targets for therapeutics. *Journal of Neurochemistry, 139*(Suppl 1), 179–197.

Bellomo, F., de Preux, F., Chung, J. P., Julien, N., Budtz-Jørgensen, E., & Müller, F. (2005). The advantages of occupational therapy in oral hygiene measures for institutionalised elderly adults. *Gerodontology, 22*(1), 24–31.

Cereda, E., Cassani, E., Barichella, M., Spadafranca, A., Caccialanza, R., Bertoli, S., et al. (2012). Low cardiometabolic risk in Parkinson's disease is independent of nutritional status, body composition and fat distribution. *Clinical Nutrition, 31*(5), 699–704.

Corcos, D. M., Lamotte, G., Luthra, N. S., & McKee, K. E. (2024). Advice to people with Parkinson's in my clinic: Exercise. *Journal of Parkinson's Disease, 14*(3), 609–617.

Fasano, A., Visanji, N. P., Liu, L. W., Lang, A. E., & Pfeiffer, R. F. (2015). Gastrointestinal dysfunction in Parkinson's disease. *Lancet Neurology, 14*(6), 625–639.

Fleming, R. E., & Ponka, P. (2012). Iron overload in human disease. *The New England Journal of Medicine, 366*(4), 348–359.

Heafield, M. T., Fearn, S., Steventon, G. B., Waring, R. H., Williams, A. C., & Sturman, S. G. (1990). Plasma cysteine and sulphate levels in patients with motor neurone. *Parkinson's and Alzheimer's disease. Neurosci Lett., 110*(1–2), 216–220.

Hosking, D. E., Eramudugolla, R., Cherbuin, N., & Anstey, K. J. (2019). MIND not Mediterranean diet related to 12-year incidence of cognitive impairment in an Australian longitudinal cohort study. *Alzheimer's & Dementia, 15*(4), 581–589.

Hu, X. W., Qin, S. M., Li, D., Hu, L. F., & Liu, C. F. (2013). Elevated homocysteine levels in levodopa-treated idiopathic Parkinson's disease: A meta-analysis. *Acta Neurologica Scandinavica, 128*(2), 73–82.

Lamberti, P., Zoccolella, S., Armenise, E., Lamberti, S. V., Fraddosio, A., de Mari, M., et al. (2005). Hyperhomocysteinemia in L-dopa treated Parkinson's disease patients: Effect of cobalamin and folate administration. *European Journal of Neurology, 12*(5), 365–368.

Lee, S. H., Kim, M. J., Kim, B. J., Kim, S. R., Chun, S., Ryu, J. S., et al. (2010). Homocysteine-lowering therapy or antioxidant therapy for bone loss in Parkinson's disease. *Movement Disorders, 25*(3), 332–340.

Lethbridge, L., Johnston, G. M., & Turnbull, G. (2013). Co-morbidities of persons dying of Parkinson's disease. *Progress Palliative Care, 21*(3), 140–145.

Metcalfe-Roach, A., Yu, A. C., Golz, E., Cirstea, M., Sundvick, K., Kliger, D., et al. (2021). MIND and Mediterranean diets associated with later onset of Parkinson's disease. *Movement Disorders, 36*(4), 977–984.

Mischley, L. K. (2017). Nutrition and nonmotor symptoms of Parkinson's disease. *International Review of Neurobiology, 134*, 1143–1161.

Molsberry, S., Bjornevik, K., Hughes, K. C., Healy, B., Schwarzschild, M., & Ascherio, A. (2020). Diet pattern and prodromal features of Parkinson disease. *Neurology, 95*(15), e2095–e2108.

Morris, H. R., Spillantini, M. G., Sue, C. M., & Williams-Gray, C. H. (2024). The pathogenesis of Parkinson's disease. *Lancet, 403*(10423), 293–304.

Postuma, R. B., Espay, A. J., Zadikoff, C., Suchowersky, O., Martin, W. R., Lafontaine, A. L., et al. (2006). Vitamins and entacapone in levodopa-induced hyperhomocysteinemia: A randomized controlled study. *Neurology, 66*(12), 1941–1943.

Rieu, I., Derost, P., Ulla, M., Marques, A., Debilly, B., De Chazeron, I., et al. (2011). Body weight gain and deep brain stimulation. *Journal of the Neurological Sciences, 310*(1–2), 267–270.

Rimmelzwaan, L. M., van Schoor, N. M., Lips, P., Berendse, H. W., & Eekhoff, E. M. (2016). Systematic review of the relationship between vitamin D and Parkinson's disease. *Journal of Parkinson's Disease, 6*(1), 29–37.

Rodrigues, B., Nóbrega, A. C., Sampaio, M., Argolo, N., & Melo, A. (2011). Silent saliva aspiration in Parkinson's disease. *Movement Disorders, 26*(1), 138–141.

Sandström, B., Davidsson, L., Eriksson, R., Alpsten, M., & Bogentoft, C. (1987). Retention of selenium (75Se), zinc (65Zn) and manganese (54Mn) in humans after intake of a labelled vitamin and mineral supplement. *Journal of Trace Elements and Electrolytes in Health and Disease, 1*(1), 33–38.

Shen, L., & Ji, H. F. (2015). Associations between vitamin D status, supplementation, outdoor work and risk of Parkinson's disease: A meta-analysis assessment. *Nutrients, 7*(6), 4817–4827.

Su, D., Cui, Y., He, C., Yin, P., Bai, R., Zhu, J., et al. (2025). Projections for prevalence of Parkinson's disease and its driving factors in 195 countries and territories to 2050: Modelling study of global burden of disease study 2021. *BMJ, 388*, e080952.

Sun, A. Y., Wang, Q., Simonyi, A., & Sun, G. Y. (2008). Botanical phenolics and brain health. *Neuromolecular Medicine, 10*(4), 259–274.

Takizawa, C., Gemmell, E., Kenworthy, J., & Speyer, R. (2016). A systematic review of the prevalence of oropharyngeal dysphagia in stroke, Parkinson's disease, Alzheimer's disease, head injury, and pneumonia. *Dysphagia, 31*(3), 434–441.

Triantafyllou, N. I., Kararizou, E., Angelopoulos, E., Tsounis, S., Boufidou, F., Evangelopoulos, M. E., et al. (2007). The influence of levodopa and the COMT inhibitor on serum vitamin B12 and folate levels in Parkinson's disease patients. *European Neurology, 58*(2), 96–99.

van den Bos, F., Speelman, A. D., Samson, M., Munneke, M., Bloem, B. R., & Verhaar, H. J. (2013). Parkinson's disease and osteoporosis. *Age and Ageing, 42*(2), 156–162.

Wu, B., Anderson, R. A., Pei, Y., Xu, H., Nye, K., Poole, P., et al. (2021). Care partner-assisted intervention to improve oral health for older adults with cognitive impairment: A feasibility study. *Gerodontology, 38*(3), 308–316.

Zhang, X., Molsberry, S. A., Schwarzschild, M. A., Ascherio, A., & Gao, X. (2022). Association of Diet and Physical Activity with all-Cause Mortality among Adults with Parkinson Disease. *JAMA Network Open, 5*(8), e2227738.

Zoccolella, S., Lamberti, P., Armenise, E., de Mari, M., Lamberti, S. V., Mastronardi, R., et al. (2005). Plasma homocysteine levels in Parkinson's disease: Role of antiparkinsonian medications. *Parkinsonism & Related Disorders, 11*(2), 131–133.

Chapter 11
Stroke

Abstract

- Stroke, caused by ischemic or hemorrhagic disruption of cerebral blood flow, is a leading cause of disability and mortality worldwide.
- Both modifiable (hypertension, diabetes, obesity, smoking, poor diet, coronary disease, inactivity, alcohol) and non-modifiable (age, sex, family history, genetics) risk factors influence stroke occurrence and outcomes.
- Nutritional challenges, including dysphagia, malnutrition, dehydration, hypermetabolism, and micronutrient deficiencies, are highly prevalent and impact recovery.
- Individualized nutritional support through oral, enteral, or parenteral routes, along with texture-modified diets and thickened liquids, is essential to reduce aspiration risk and optimize intake.
- Dietary patterns such as Mediterranean, DASH, MIND, Nordic, and other plant-based diets support recovery and reduce recurrent stroke risk.
- Targeted nutrients including magnesium, potassium, calcium, selenium, vitamins B6, B12, folate, C, D, E, K, choline, fiber, and omega-3 fatty acids (EPA/DHA) are critical for prevention and rehabilitation.
- Caution with supplementation is required; avoid excessive calcium and vitamin E, routine antioxidants are not recommended, and niacin with statins may increase mortality risk.
- Early enteral nutrition is recommended for prolonged dysphagia, with parenteral nutrition as needed; EPA/DHA-enriched formulas may offer additional benefits.
- Consideration of food–drug interactions is essential to optimize recovery, reduce complications, and support rehabilitation.

Keywords Stroke · Malnutrition · Nutrition · Micronutrients · Trace elements · Dietary patterns · Enteral nutrition · Parenteral nutrition · Supplementation · Food–drug interactions

M. H. Rouhani et al., *The Healing Plate*, SpringerBriefs in Modern Perspectives on Disability Research, https://doi.org/10.1007/978-981-95-8150-4_11

11.1 Definition and Epidemiology

Stroke is not only an acute neurological event but also one of the most disabling disorders worldwide, characterized by a sudden interruption of cerebral blood flow, resulting in rapid neuronal injury, hypoxia-induced necrosis, and frequently irreversible neurological deficits (American Heart Association Statistics Committee and Stroke Statistics Subcommittee, 2017). Beyond its acute phase, stroke is universally recognized as a leading cause of long-term disability, leaving millions of survivors with persistent motor, sensory, cognitive, and speech impairments that severely compromise independence and quality of life. Strokes are classified into ischemic and hemorrhagic (American Heart Association Statistics Committee and Stroke Statistics Subcommittee, 2017; Siow et al., 2021). Globally, stroke is the second leading cause of death and the third major contributor to Disability-Adjusted Life Years (DALYs) (World Health Organization, 2020). In the United States alone, the annual economic burden of stroke is estimated at $34 billion, encompassing direct medical costs, pharmaceutical expenses, and indirect losses related to disability. Thus, stroke stands as both a critical acute medical emergency and one of the foremost chronic disability disorders.

11.2 Etiology

Stroke, or cerebrovascular accident, occurs either due to sudden interruption of cerebral blood flow (ischemic stroke, ~87% of cases) or rupture of a brain vessel (hemorrhagic stroke), leading to rapid neuronal death (Benjamin et al., 2017). Ischemic strokes result from either thrombotic event, where a blood clot forms locally often due to atherosclerosis, arterial dissection, fibromuscular dysplasia, or inflammation; or embolic events, where circulating debris from the heart or proximal arteries occludes cerebral vessels; occasionally, emboli pass through right-to-left shunts such as a patent foramen ovale. Hemorrhagic strokes arise from vascular rupture and are less common but more lethal. Severe strokes are often preceded by transient ischemic attacks (TIAs), which are short-lived episodes of reduced blood flow to the brain that cause temporary neurological symptoms but leave no lasting damage (Lui et al., 2025). Etiology critically influences prognosis and outcomes (Ntaios, 2020; Pierik et al., 2020), guiding monitoring and management strategies for coagulation and inflammation, especially in patients with risk factors such as advanced age, hypertension, smoking, poor diet, obesity, coronary heart disease, diabetes, physical inactivity, alcohol intake, and genetic predisposition.

11.3 Nutritional Management

11.3.1 Nutritional Challenges

Malnutrition and dehydration are highly prevalent among stroke patients, primarily due to dysphagia, impaired consciousness, cognitive dysfunction, and perception deficits (Gomes et al., 2016). Poor nutritional status, either pre-stroke or at admission, is strongly linked to increased 30-day mortality, higher complication rates, and poorer outcomes (Gomes et al., 2016; Bell et al., 2014; Bell et al., 2013). Nutritional deterioration commonly progresses within the first week post-stroke (FOOD Trial Collaboration, 2003; Yoo et al., 2008).

Additional contributors include hypermetabolism in the acute phase, inability to swallow, comatose states, and metabolic alterations such as impaired protein synthesis, oxidative stress, and zinc deficiency (Aquilani et al., 2008; Aquilani et al., 2010; Aquilani et al., 2009). Since most cognitive recovery occurs within the first 30 days, early detection and management of dysphagia and immediate initiation of individualized nutritional support including oral, enteral, parenteral, or combined are critical (Aquilani et al., 2011). Persistent nutrition-related challenges during rehabilitation necessitate ongoing monitoring and tailored interventions to optimize functional recovery and reduce complications.

11.3.2 General Dietary Recommendations

Nutrition is a cornerstone in both preventing stroke and optimizing recovery after its occurrence, primarily by modulating key risk factors including hypertension, atherosclerosis, diabetes, and systemic inflammation. Diets rich in fruits, vegetables, whole grains, nuts, seeds, legumes, low-fat dairy, and fatty fish, with limited intake of red and processed meats, refined carbohydrates, added sugars, and excessive sodium, demonstrate strong protective effects (Hankey, 2017). Emerging evidence indicates that greater adherence to plant-based dietary patterns, including the Mediterranean, DASH, Mind, prudent, and Nordic diets, is associated with a reduced risk of stroke (Hankey, 2017; Hankey, 2012; English et al., 2021; Sherzai et al., 2012). Nuts (20–30 g/day) indicated beneficial effects in reduced stroke incidence through endothelial function improvements and oxidative stress and inflammation reduction. Similarly, moderate intake of dark chocolate, rich in flavonoids and polyphenols, has been associated with a reduced risk of total stroke. Moreover, a diet emphasizing low-glycemic load (GL) carbohydrates and prioritizing whole grains is recommended to mitigate stroke risk. In addition to avoiding trans fatty acids, replacing saturated fats and refined carbohydrates with sources rich in Monounsaturated Fatty Acids (MUFAs) and Polyunsaturated Fatty Acids (PUFAs), such as extra virgin olive oil, nuts, seeds, and fatty fish, further enhances long-term cardiometabolic health. Regular consumption of omega-3–rich fatty fish (twice weekly) elevates serum Docosahexaenoic Acid (DHA) levels and is associated with a reduced risk of stroke, whereas omega-3 supplements provide inconsistent benefits and may be unsafe in patients taking anticoagulants (e.g., warfarin, aspirin) (National Institutes of Health: National Center for Complimentary and Integrative Health (NCCIH): Omega-3 supplements: an introduction, 2013; Saber et al., 2017). Epidemiological evidence suggests that higher fish intake is associated with a lower risk of total and ischemic stroke (no consistent association with hemorrhagic stroke). Additionally, regular consumption of low-fat dairy supplies calcium, magnesium, potassium, and bioactive peptides with protective effects against both ischemic and hemorrhagic stroke. In contrast, frequent intake of red and especially processed meats correlates with increased total and ischemic stroke incidence (Kaluza et al., 2013). Limiting sugar-sweetened beverages is also critical. Moreover, moderate coffee and tea especially green tea consumption has been linked to a reduced risk of total and ischemic stroke through its polyphenols and chlorogenic acid with antioxidant and anti-inflammatory actions.

11.3.3 Targeted Nutrients and Supplements

Magnesium: Adequate magnesium intake reduces stroke risk by regulating blood pressure, improving insulin sensitivity, and optimizing lipid metabolism.

Potassium: Its protective benefits are especially pronounced when sodium intake is high, emphasizing the importance of maintaining an appropriate potassium-to-sodium balance for both stroke prevention and hypertension management.

Sodium: Excess sodium is an independent risk factor for stroke, and renal disease. Reducing daily sodium intake from ~3200–4000 mg (≈8–10 g salt) to <2300 mg/day (<6 g salt) can reduce stroke risk (Snetselaar et al., 2021; Ma et al., 2022).

Calcium: Adequate calcium intake may lower stroke risk by reducing hypertension and systemic inflammation, especially in overweight individuals.

Selenium: Evidence indicates that this trace element can enhance neurological recovery after intracerebral hemorrhage by upregulating Glutathione Peroxidase 4 (GPX4), limiting neuronal cell death, and improving functional outcomes; however, its routine clinical application has not yet been established (Alim et al., 2019).

B Vitamins: Adequate intake of folate, vitamin B6, and vitamin B12 is essential for stroke prevention, primarily by lowering homocysteine and reducing oxidative stress. Folic acid supplementation, alone or with low-dose B12, is most effective in individuals with low baseline folate, while benefits are limited in those with established cardiovascular disease or prior stroke (Zhao et al., 2017; Hsu et al.,

2018; Christen et al., 2018; Toole et al., 2004; Wang et al., 2007). Older adults choosing supplementation are advised to limit folic acid to ≤400 μg/day, keeping total intake below the upper limit of 1000 μg/day (Saposnik et al., 2009).

Vitamin C: Adequate vitamin C intake reduces stroke risk by preventing endothelial dysfunction, exerting anti-inflammatory effects, and lowering blood pressure.

Vitamin D: Normal serum vitamin D may lower stroke risk by improving blood pressure, insulin sensitivity, endothelial function, and vascular smooth muscle regulation.

Vitamin K: Vitamin K could help reduce vascular calcification, and a daily intake of 500 μg might be required.

Vitamin E: Intake above the Estimated Average Requirement (EAR) may support immune function and reduce inflammation (Meydani et al., 2018), but long-term α-tocopherol supplementation at 50–180 mg/day can increase hemorrhagic stroke risk (National Institutes of Health, Office of Dietary Supplements, Vitamin E, 2021).

Choline: Adequate choline intake (550 mg/day for men, 450 mg/day for women, and 550 mg/day during lactation) plays a potential neuroprotective role in stroke.

Dietary fiber: Adequate fiber intake (≥25 g/day) reduces stroke risk by improving blood pressure, insulin sensitivity, lipid metabolism, and endothelial function.

Omega-3 fatty acids: Supplementation with Eicosapentaenoic Acid (EPA) and DHA, via fish oil or purified icosapent ethyl, has demonstrated significant benefits for ischemic stroke prevention and cardiovascular risk reduction. The FDA has approved icosapent ethyl 4 g/day as an adjunct to maximally tolerated statin therapy to lower major cardiovascular events, including stroke, in adults with elevated triglycerides (>150 mg/dL) and high cardiovascular risk. For general supplementation, 1–4 g/day of combined EPA + DHA is effective, with up to 3 g/day recognized as safe (GRAS); the FDA recommends ≤2 g/day from supplements.

11.3.4 Caution in Supplement Prescribing

Calcium: Supplementation should be reserved for confirmed deficiencies due to potential increased risk of cerebrovascular and cardiovascular events, particularly in postmenopausal women; excessive intake may disrupt vascular homeostasis and promote calcification or thrombosis.

Vitamin E: High intake, whether dietary or supplemental, is associated with an increased risk of hemorrhagic stroke.

Antioxidant Vitamins: Routine use of antioxidant vitamin supplements for stroke prevention is not recommended.

Niacin: Co-administration of niacin with statin therapy has been linked to increased all-cause mortality and should be used cautiously.

11.3.5 Enteral and Parenteral Nutrition

Early enteral nutrition (EN) is strongly recommended for stroke patients with anticipated prolonged dysphagia (>7 days) or insufficient oral intake, ideally initiated within 24–72 h of admission when the gastrointestinal tract is functional (McClave et al., 2016). During the acute phase, nasogastric tube feeding is preferred and does not hinder dysphagia rehabilitation; a nasal bridle may be used in case of repeated dislodgement. For long-term needs (>28 days), percutaneous endoscopic gastrostomy (PEG) should be placed during a stable clinical phase (after 14–28 days) (Burgos et al., 2018). Furthermore, in mechanically ventilated patients, particularly those ventilated for >48 h, early PEG (within 1 week) may lower the risk of ventilation-associated pneumonia (Kostadima et al., 2005; Braunschweig et al., 2001). Dysphagia resolves within 7–14 days in most ischemic stroke patients; thus, less invasive access than PEG is often sufficient initially (Peschl et al., 1988; Gordon et al., 1987; Smithard et al., 1997). Continuous monitoring of tube position and early initiation of dysphagia therapy are essential. Thickened liquids can reduce aspiration risk in oropharyngeal dysphagia but may increase post-swallow residue, requiring individualized management (Burgos et al., 2018). Immunomodulating EN formulas enriched with EPA and DHA, as recommended for traumatic brain injury, may also benefit acute stroke patients with increased metabolic demands (McClave et al., 2016). Routine oral nutritional supplementation (ONS) is not indicated for well-nourished, non-dysphagic patients, as it does not improve survival or functional outcomes, but may be beneficial in those with diagnosed malnutrition (Wirth et al., 2013; Geeganage et al., 2012). Parenteral nutrition (PN) should be considered if EN is not tolerated or fails to meet nutritional requirements. Overall, evidence strongly supports the early initiation of individualized enteral or parenteral nutrition as a cornerstone of acute stroke care to meet metabolic needs, prevent malnutrition, and facilitate recovery and rehabilitation.

11.3.6 Recommendation

In stroke patients, particularly those with dysphagia, timely nutritional intervention is essential to prevent complications and optimize recovery. Texture-modified diets and thickened liquids can reduce aspiration and choking risk and may lower aspiration pneumonia incidence; however, they often decrease overall energy and fluid intake, necessitating individualized monitoring by trained professionals. Strategies such as supervised free water protocols, cautious provision of un-thickened water in selected patients, and the use of carbonated liquids to reduce pharyngeal residue may enhance both safety and nutritional adequacy.

11.4 Food–Drug Interactions

Although pharmacotherapy is indispensable in both the acute treatment and long-term secondary prevention of stroke, optimal outcomes are highly dependent on dietary considerations. Food–drug interactions may alter the pharmacokinetics and pharmacodynamics of commonly prescribed medications, thereby influencing their efficacy, safety, and tolerability. Key pharmacological classes include thrombolytics, antiplatelet agents, anticoagulants, antihypertensives, and lipid-lowering therapies (Lip et al., 2022; Yoshimura, 2024). The most common medication that are used in stroke along with their food–drug interaction is illustrated in Table 11.1.

Table 11.1 Commonly prescribed medications for stroke and their food–drug interactions

Drug	Trade name	Food–drug interactions
Antiplatelet		
Clopidogrel	Plavix	Side effects: Diarrhea, gastric, or peptic ulcer, gastritis, nausea and vomiting, stomach pain Avoid: Garlic, grapefruit
Aspirin	Bayer	Side effects: Weight gain, nausea or vomiting, diarrhea, constipation, severe GI irritation (bleeding, gastritis, ulceration), nutrient depletions (hypokalemia, iron-folic acid—Vitamin C—Vitamin E deficiencies), dyspepsia, bezoar formation, loss of appetite, upset stomach, hypoglycemia (by taking high doses) Avoid: Caffeine, alcohol, omega-3 fatty acids, chromium
Ticagrelor	Brilique	Side effects: Nausea or vomiting, diarrhea, constipation, bleeding Avoid: Grapefruit
Anticoagulant		
Warfarin	Coumadin	Side effects: Increased risk of bleeding, hypoglycemia Avoid: Alcohol, St. John's wort, Omega-3 fatty acids, CoQ10, vitamin K rich foods include beef liver, broccoli, Brussels sprouts, cabbage, collard greens, endive, kale, lettuce, mustard greens, parsley, soybeans, spinach, Swiss chard, turnip greens, watercress, asparagus, avocados, dill pickles, green peas, green tea, canola oil, margarine, mayonnaise, olive oil, soybean oil, and herbal products such as dong quai, ginseng * when taking these medications, it is necessary to eat a normal, balanced diet, maintaining a consistent amount of vitamin K, and avoiding drastic changes in dietary habits. *interrupt enteral feeding 1 h before and after warfarin; avoid soy protein-based formulas

(continued)

Table 11.1 (continued)

Drug	Trade name	Food–drug interactions
Heparin	Hep-lock	Side effects: Bleeding, abdominal pain or swelling, nausea or vomiting, diarrhea, or constipation Avoid: Alcohol, garlic, ginger, ginseng, ginkgo, cannabis, saw palmetto, green tea, papaya, mango or onion, vitamin K-rich foods include beef liver, broccoli, Brussels sprouts, cabbage, collard greens, endive, kale, lettuce, mustard greens, parsley, soybeans, spinach, Swiss chard, turnip greens, watercress, asparagus, avocados, dill pickles, green peas, green tea, canola oil, margarine, mayonnaise, olive oil, soybean oil
Rivaroxaban	Xarelto	Side effects: Increase calcium loss, bleeding, nausea, or vomiting Avoid: Alcohol, grapefruit, St. John's wort
Thrombolytic		
Alteplase	Activase	Side effects: Swallowing difficulty Avoid: Alcohol, and agents with anticoagulant/antiplatelet activity; examples include garlic, ginger, bilberry, danshen, and ginkgo biloba
Tenecteplase	TNKase	Side effects: Swallowing difficulty, constipation, diarrhea, nausea, thirst, vomiting Avoid: -
HMG-CoA reductase inhibitor		
Atorvastatin	Lipitor	Side effects: Nausea, diarrhea, constipation Avoid: Grapefruit, high-fiber diets
ACE inhibitors		
Captopril	Capoten	Side effects: Causes dysgeusia (metallic or salty taste) and the loss of taste perception, induce hypoglycemic events, stomach pain Avoid: Grapefruit, high potassium dietary intakes, and potassium salt substitutes
Angiotensin II receptor blockers (ARBs)		
Losartan	Cozaar	Side effects: Diarrhea, nausea, vomiting, hyperkalemia, hyponatremia Avoid: High-potassium diet, potassium-containing salt substitutes, alcohol
Beta-blocker		
Metoprolol	Toprol XL	Side effects: Constipation, diarrhea, hepatitis, nausea, and vomiting Avoid: Alcohol, natural licorice, and multivitamin minerals
Calcium Channel blockers (CCBs)		
Diltiazem		Side effects: Constipation, stomach pain Avoid: Grapefruit, natural licorice, alcohol, ginkgo, fumitory, hawthorn, khella, calcium, or vitamin D in large doses
Diuretics		
Furosemide	Lasix	Side effects: Causes nutrient depletions (hypocalcemia, hypokalemia, hypomagnesemia) Avoid: Alcohol
Hydrochlorothiazide	Esidrix	Side effects: Causes nutrient depletions (hypomagnesemia, hypokalemia, zinc deficiency) Avoid: High-carbohydrate meals, sodium in foods, alcohol
Metolazone	Zaroxolyn	Side effects: - Avoid: Alcohol

Acknowledgments The authors confirm that the content, analysis, and conclusions of this manuscript are their own work. AI-based tools were used solely to assist in improving the clarity and correctness of the English language.

References

Alim, I., Caulfield, J. T., Chen, Y., Swarup, V., Geschwind, D. H., Ivanova, E., et al. (2019). Selenium drives a transcriptional adaptive program to block Ferroptosis and treat stroke. *Cell, 177*(5), 1262–1279.e25.

American Heart Association Statistics Committee and Stroke Statistics Subcommittee. (2017). Heart disease and stroke statistics—2017 update: A report from the american heart association. *Circulation, 135*, e229–e445.

Aquilani, R., Baiardi, P., Scocchi, M., Iadarola, P., Verri, M., Sessarego, P., et al. (2009). Normalization of zinc intake enhances neurological retrieval of patients suffering from ischemic strokes. *Nutritional Neuroscience, 12*(5), 219–225.

Aquilani, R., Scocchi, M., Boschi, F., Viglio, S., Iadarola, P., Pastoris, O., et al. (2008). Effect of calorie-protein supplementation on the cognitive recovery of patients with subacute stroke. *Nutritional Neuroscience, 11*(5), 235–240.

Aquilani, R., Scocchi, M., Iadarola, P., Viglio, S., Pasini, E., Condello, S., et al. (2010). Spontaneous neurocognitive retrieval of patients with sub-acute ischemic stroke is associated with dietary protein intake. *Nutritional Neuroscience, 13*(3), 129–134.

Aquilani, R., Sessarego, P., Iadarola, P., Barbieri, A., & Boschi, F. (2011). Nutrition for brain recovery after ischemic stroke: An added value to rehabilitation. *Nutrition in Clinical Practice, 26*(3), 339–345.

Bell, C. L., LaCroix, A., Masaki, K., Hade, E. M., Manini, T., Mysiw, W. J., et al. (2013). Prestroke factors associated with poststroke mortality and recovery in older women in the Women's Health Initiative. *Journal of the American Geriatrics Society, 61*(8), 1324–1330.

Bell, C. L., Rantanen, T., Chen, R., Davis, J., Petrovitch, H., Ross, G. W., et al. (2014). Prestroke weight loss is associated with poststroke mortality among men in the Honolulu-Asia aging study. *Archives of Physical Medicine and Rehabilitation, 95*(3), 472–479.

Benjamin, E. J., Blaha, M. J., Chiuve, S. E., Cushman, M., Das, S. R., Deo, R., et al. (2017). Heart disease and stroke Statistics-2017 update: A report from the American Heart Association. *Circulation, 135*(10), e146–e603.

Braunschweig, C. L., Levy, P., Sheean, P. M., & Wang, X. (2001). Enteral compared with parenteral nutrition: A meta-analysis. *The American Journal of Clinical Nutrition, 74*(4), 534–542.

Burgos, R., Bretón, I., Cereda, E., Desport, J. C., Dziewas, R., Genton, L., et al. (2018). ESPEN guideline clinical nutrition in neurology. *Clinical Nutrition, 37*(1), 354–396.

Christen, W. G., Cook, N. R., Van Denburgh, M., Zaharris, E., Albert, C. M., & Manson, J. E. (2018). Effect of combined treatment with folic acid, vitamin B(6), and vitamin B(12) on plasma biomarkers of inflammation and endothelial dysfunction in women. *Journal of the American Heart Association, 7*(11), e008517.

English, C., MacDonald-Wicks, L., Patterson, A., Attia, J., & Hankey, G. J. (2021). The role of diet in secondary stroke prevention. *Lancet Neurology, 20*(2), 150–160.

FOOD Trial Collaboration. (2003). Poor nutritional status on admission predicts poor outcomes after stroke: Observational data from the FOOD trial. *Stroke, 34*(6), 1450–1456.

Geeganage, C., Beavan, J., Ellender, S., & Bath, P. M. (2012). Interventions for dysphagia and nutritional support in acute and subacute stroke. *Cochrane Database of Systematic Reviews, 10*, Cd000323.

Gomes, F., Emery, P. W., & Weekes, C. E. (2016). Risk of malnutrition is an independent predictor of mortality, length of hospital stay, and hospitalization costs in stroke patients. *Journal of Stroke and Cerebrovascular Diseases, 25*(4), 799–806.

Gordon, C., Hewer, R. L., & Wade, D. T. (1987). Dysphagia in acute stroke. *British Medical Journal (Clinical Research Ed.), 295*(6595), 411–414.

Hankey, G. J. (2012). Nutrition and the risk of stroke. *Lancet Neurology, 11*(1), 66–81.

Hankey, G. J. (2017). The role of nutrition in the risk and burden of stroke: An update of the evidence. *Stroke, 48*(11), 3168–3174.

Hsu, C. Y., Chiu, S. W., Hong, K. S., Saver, J. L., Wu, Y. L., Lee, J. D., et al. (2018). Folic acid in stroke prevention in countries without mandatory folic acid food fortification: A meta-analysis of randomized controlled trials. *J Stroke., 20*(1), 99–109.

Kaluza, J., Wolk, A., & Larsson, S. C. (2013). Heme iron intake and risk of stroke: A prospective study of men. *Stroke, 44*(2), 334–339.

Kostadima, E., Kaditis, A. G., Alexopoulos, E. I., Zakynthinos, E., & Sfyras, D. (2005). Early gastrostomy reduces the rate of ventilator-associated pneumonia in stroke or head injury patients. *The European Respiratory Journal, 26*(1), 106–111.

Lip, G. Y. H., Lane, D. A., Lenarczyk, R., Boriani, G., Doehner, W., Benjamin, L. A., et al. (2022). Integrated care for optimizing the management of stroke and associated heart disease: A position paper of the European Society of Cardiology Council on stroke. *European Heart Journal, 43*(26), 2442–2460.

Lui, F., Khan Suheb, M. Z., & Patti, L. (2025). *Ischemic stroke*. StatPearls. Treasure Island (FL): StatPearls Publishing Copyright © 2025, StatPearls Publishing LLC.

Ma, Y., He, F. J., Sun, Q., Yuan, C., Kieneker, L. M., Curhan, G. C., et al. (2022). 24-hour urinary sodium and potassium excretion and cardiovascular risk. *The New England Journal of Medicine, 386*(3), 252–263.

McClave, S. A., Taylor, B. E., Martindale, R. G., Warren, M. M., Johnson, D. R., Braunschweig, C., et al. (2016). Guidelines for the provision and assessment of nutrition support therapy in the adult critically ill patient. *Journal of Parenteral and Enteral Nutrition, 40*(2), 159–211.

Meydani, S. N., Lewis, E. D., & Wu, D. (2018). Perspective: Should vitamin E recommendations for older adults be increased? *Advances in Nutrition, 9*(5), 533–543.

National Institutes of Health, Office of Dietary Supplements, Vitamin E. (2021). Retrieved June 28, 2022, from https://ods.od.nih.gov/factsheets/VitaminE-HealthProfessional

National Institutes of Health: National Center for Complimentary and Integrative Health (NCCIH). (2013). *Omega-3 supplements: An introduction.* https://nccih.nih.gov/health/omega3/introduction.htm

Ntaios, G. (2020). Embolic stroke of undetermined source: JACC review topic of the week. *Journal of the American College of Cardiology, 75*(3), 333–340.

Peschl, L., Zeilinger, M., Munda, W., Prem, H., & Schragel, D. (1988). Percutaneous endoscopic gastrostomy—a possibility for enteral feeding of patients with severe cerebral dysfunctions. *Wiener Klinische Wochenschrift, 100*(10), 314–318.

Pierik, R., Algra, A., van Dijk, E., Erasmus, M. E., van Gelder, I. C., Koudstaal, P. J., et al. (2020). Distribution of Cardioembolic stroke: A cohort study. *Cerebrovascular Diseases, 49*(1), 97–104.

Saber, H., Yakoob, M. Y., Shi, P., Longstreth, W. T., Jr., Lemaitre, R. N., Siscovick, D., et al. (2017). Omega-3 fatty acids and incident ischemic stroke and its Atherothrombotic and Cardioembolic subtypes in 3 US cohorts. *Stroke, 48*(10), 2678–2685.

Saposnik, G., Ray, J. G., Sheridan, P., McQueen, M., & Lonn, E. (2009). Homocysteine-lowering therapy and stroke risk, severity, and disability: Additional findings from the HOPE 2 trial. *Stroke, 40*(4), 1365–1372.

Sherzai, A., Heim, L. T., Boothby, C., & Sherzai, A. D. (2012). Stroke, food groups, and dietary patterns: A systematic review. *Nutrition Reviews, 70*(8), 423–435.

Siow, I., Lee, K. S., Zhang, J. J. Y., Saffari, S. E., Ng, A., & Young, B. (2021). Stroke as a neurological complication of COVID-19: A systematic review and meta-analysis of incidence, outcomes and predictors. *Journal of Stroke and Cerebrovascular Diseases, 30*(3), 105549.

Smithard, D. G., O'Neill, P. A., England, R. E., Park, C. L., Wyatt, R., Martin, D. F., et al. (1997). The natural history of dysphagia following a stroke. *Dysphagia, 12*(4), 188–193.

Snetselaar, L. G., de Jesus, J. M., DeSilva, D. M., & Stoody, E. E. (2021). Dietary guidelines for Americans, 2020–2025: Understanding the scientific process, guidelines, and key recommendations. *Nutrition Today, 56*(6), 287–295.

Toole, J. F., Malinow, M. R., Chambless, L. E., Spence, J. D., Pettigrew, L. C., Howard, V. J., et al. (2004). Lowering homocysteine in patients with ischemic stroke to prevent recurrent stroke, myocardial infarction, and death: The vitamin intervention for stroke prevention (VISP) randomized controlled trial. *Journal of the American Medical Association, 291*(5), 565–575.

Wang, X., Qin, X., Demirtas, H., Li, J., Mao, G., Huo, Y., et al. (2007). Efficacy of folic acid supplementation in stroke prevention: A meta-analysis. *Lancet, 369*(9576), 1876–1882.

Wirth, R., Smoliner, C., Jäger, M., Warnecke, T., Leischker, A. H., & Dziewas, R. (2013). Guideline clinical nutrition in patients with stroke. *Experimental & Translational Stroke Medicine, 5*(1), 14.

World Health Organization. (2020). *Global health estimates: Life expectancy and leading causes of death and disability*. https://www.who.int/data/gho/data/themes/mortalityandglobalhealthestimates

Yoo, S. H., Kim, J. S., Kwon, S. U., Yun, S. C., Koh, J. Y., & Kang, D. W. (2008). Undernutrition as a predictor of poor clinical outcomes in acute ischemic stroke patients. *Archives of Neurology, 65*(1), 39–43.

Yoshimura, S. (2024). Medical Management of Acute Stroke based on Japan stroke society guidelines and the Japan stroke data Bank. *Journal of Atherosclerosis and Thrombosis, 31*(12), 1652–1659.

Zhao, M., Wu, G., Li, Y., Wang, X., Hou, F. F., Xu, X., et al. (2017). Meta-analysis of folic acid efficacy trials in stroke prevention: Insight into effect modifiers. *Neurology, 88*(19), 1830–1838.

Chapter 12
Multiple Sclerosis

Abstract

- Multiple sclerosis (MS) is a chronic autoimmune disease of the central nervous system, causing fatigue, spasticity, tremor, pain, visual and sensory deficits, muscle weakness, bladder/bowel dysfunction, and cognitive decline.
- MS affects ~1.89 million people worldwide, with women nearly twice as likely as men to be diagnosed, particularly between ages 15–40.
- Risk factors include genetic susceptibility, viral infections (e.g., EBV), low vitamin D, smoking, obesity, and low sun exposure.
- Nutritional management is a key complementary strategy, addressing bowel dysfunction, malnutrition, high-calorie intake, and weight management to improve quality of life.
- Dietary approaches studied include Mediterranean, Paleolithic, Swank, McDougall, Ketogenic, caloric restriction, intermittent fasting, and gluten-free diets; these may reduce inflammation, modulate gut microbiota, and improve fatigue.
- Macronutrient recommendations: plant-based protein, high-fiber carbohydrates with limited simple sugars (<10% energy), and low-saturated-fat diets emphasizing MUFAs/PUFAs; omega-3/fish oil may reduce relapse rates.
- Micronutrients: vitamins D, A, E, K, B-complex, calcium, potassium, and selenium are important; deficiencies are common and may affect disease activity.
- Pharmacological management targets symptom relief with immunomodulators (glatiramer acetate, interferons), antispasticity agents (baclofen, tizanidine), corticosteroids (methylprednisolone), stimulants (amantadine, modafinil), anticonvulsants (gabapentin, carbamazepine), and antidepressants (amitriptyline, sertraline, fluoxetine), considering side effects and food–drug interactions.

Keywords Multiple sclerosis (MS) · Central nervous system (CNS) · Autoimmune disorder · Nutritional management · Dietary patterns · Macronutrients · Micronutrients · Pharmacological treatments · Food · Drug interactions

M. H. Rouhani et al., *The Healing Plate*, SpringerBriefs in Modern Perspectives on Disability Research, https://doi.org/10.1007/978-981-95-8150-4_12

12.1 Definition and Epidemiology

Multiple sclerosis (MS) is a long-lasting autoimmune disorder of the central nervous system (CNS), marked by inflammation, myelin damage, gliosis, and progressive neuronal loss. This disorder presents with diverse neurological manifestations, including visual disturbances, sensory deficits like numbness and tingling, localized muscle weakness, bladder and bowel dysfunction, and cognitive decline (Tafti et al., 2025). Epidemiological evidence indicates that MS affects about 1.89 million people worldwide. The global prevalence is estimated at 23.9 cases per 100,000 population, and this rate has shown a steady rise over the past three decades. Women are nearly twice as likely to be diagnosed with MS compared to men, particularly within the 15–40-year age group (Khan & Hashim, 2025).

12.2 Etiology

It is currently believed that MS arises from a combination of genetic susceptibility and environmental influences, although its precise cause has not yet been identified. Genetic predisposition plays a role in a minority of cases (Raymond, 2023). Environmental factors from early life through young adulthood appear to contribute significantly to disease onset (Haki et al., 2024). Epidemiologic evidence indicates that geographic latitude and sun exposure influence MS risk; individuals living in regions with lower sunlight, which may lead to vitamin D deficiency, show a higher incidence (Langer-Gould et al., 2018; Simpson Jr. et al., 2018; Zahoor & Haq, 2017). Viral infections, particularly Epstein-Barr virus, have been identified as environmental risk factors for MS, and human herpesvirus 6 is under investigation for its potential role in triggering relapses (Fernández-Menéndez et al., 2016; Society NMS, n.d.-a). Additionally, lifestyle factors such as smoking and obesity in childhood or adolescence, especially in females, have been linked to increased MS risk and more severe disease progression (Novo & Batista, 2017; Society NMS, n.d.-b).

12.3 Nutritional Management

Nutrition plays a crucial role in the management of MS, a chronic inflammatory and immune-mediated disease of the CNS. Although pharmacological therapies are essential for disease control, they are not always sufficient to halt disease progression (Filippini et al., 2013; Bridel & Lalive, 2014; Loleit et al., 2014). Dietary interventions are increasingly recognized as a low-risk, complementary approach to improve clinical outcomes, well-being, and quality of life (QOL) in MS patients (Penesová et al., 2018).

12.3.1 Nutritional Challenges

Patients with MS encounter several nutritional difficulties that may worsen disease progression or symptom burden. Increased intestinal permeability in MS allows large amounts of dietary lectins to damage the gut lining, leading to higher permeability. Nightshade vegetables (potatoes, tomatoes, eggplant, peppers) may exacerbate autoimmune responses due to lectins and alkaloids and are often limited in elimination-style diets (Vojdani, 2015). This, in turn, enables bacterial fragments such as lipopolysaccharide and incompletely digested food proteins to enter the bloodstream, potentially triggering immune responses that contribute to disease activity (Buscarinu et al., 2018). Bowel dysfunction is also highly prevalent. Constipation and fecal incontinence may coexist and alternate, severely affecting patients' QOL and social interactions, while simultaneously burdening caregivers and increasing healthcare costs (Preziosi et al., 2018). Moreover, overconsumption of high-calorie foods and obesity can accelerate disease progression and increase the risk of brain volume loss, highlighting the importance of careful energy balance (Ghadirian et al., 1998; Mohammadi et al., 2024; Mowry et al., 2018).

12.3.2 General Dietary Recommendations

While no diet has definitive evidence for MS management, the National MS Society recommend adherence to general healthy eating principles, such as those outlined in the U.S. Dietary Guidelines for Americans (DGA) and guidelines for cancer and cardiovascular disease prevention (Agriculture UDoHaHSUDo, 2015; Eckel et al., 2014; Society NMS, n.d.-c).

12.3.3 Dietary Patterns

Dietary approaches have been studied in order to improve outcomes in MS. Although no approach is definitively proven, several studies suggest that eating habits may influence the disease course. The most commonly explored diets include the Mediterranean, Paleolithic, Swank, McDougall, and Hypercaloric restriction, Ketogenic, and Gluten-free diets (Penesová et al., 2018; Altowaijri et al., 2017).

Mediterranean Diet: The Mediterranean diet emphasizes high consumption of fruits, vegetables, whole grains, and olive oil as the main fat source, with moderate intake of fish and dairy and limited red meat (Katz, 2018). Olive oil phenols exert anti-inflammatory effects and protect against oxidative stress. Studies suggest that this diet reduces inflammatory markers (Altowaijri et al., 2017; Wiseman et al., 2002), regulates vascular risk factors, modulates gut microbiota (Santangelo et al., 2018; Evans et al., 2019), and is associated with lower MS onset risk (Bronzini et al., 2024).

Paleolithic Diet: This diet is rich in leafy green vegetables, plant proteins, soy, and nuts, while it is poor in legumes, dairy products, sugar, processed foods, oils, and foods containing gluten such as grains, and includes a moderate intake of meats (Irish et al., 2017; Stoiloudis et al., 2022). Clinical observations reported reduced fatigue in MS patients, although nutritional deficiencies remain a concern (Stoiloudis et al., 2022).

Swank Diet: The Swank diet is characterized by restricted saturated fatty acids (SFAs) and processed foods with emphasis on fruits, vegetables, and unsaturated fats. Long-term adherence was associated with significant reductions in fatigue and improvements in QOL (Wahls et al., 2021).

McDougall Diet: This plant-based diet relies heavily on carbohydrates, avoiding oils, animal products, eggs, and dairy. Some studies reported reduced fatigue in MS patients, though no significant effects on clinical relapse rates (Katz, 2018).

Caloric Restriction and Intermittent Fasting: Excess caloric intake may promote inflammation (Kökten et al., 2021). Caloric restriction has the ability to modulate the immune, inflammatory, and metabolic profiles while counteracting some of the key pathogenic mechanisms underlying the disease (Ghezzi et al., 2025). Intermittent fasting is being investigated as complementary strategy in MS management, with evidence suggesting potential benefits in reducing inflammation and promoting neuroprotection (Koukach et al., 2025).

Ketogenic Diet: The ketogenic diet is high-fat and low-carbohydrate, inducing ketone production with anti-inflammatory potential. Trials suggest improvements in fatigue, depression, neurological disability, and QOL, though risks include vitamin deficiencies, weight loss, and gastrointestinal symptoms (Choi et al., 2016; Cordain, 2018; de la Rubia Ortí et al., 2023; Skartun et al., 2025).

Gluten-free Diet: Evidence for gluten-free diets in MS is limited. Some studies reported improvements in Expanded Disability Status Scale, lesion activity, fatigue, and QOL, but results remain inconsistent due to bias and lack of randomized controlled trials (Thomsen et al., 2019).

12.3.4 Energy and Macronutrients Requirements

Caloric Intake: Both underweight and overweight conditions can pose risks in MS, underscoring the importance of balanced energy intake.

Weight Loss: If energy needs are low due to reduced activity or eating difficulties, weight loss may occur, leading to malnutrition. Signs include fatigue and muscle weakness, which overlap with MS symptoms. High-energy supplements (available over-the-counter or on prescription) are recommended, taken between meals to boost calories. Fortifying foods (e.g., adding extra calories via full-fat products) is also advised.

Weight Gain: Reduced mobility or certain treatments (e.g., steroids) can lower energy expenditure, leading to excess weight. Strategies include monitoring fluid choices (e.g., avoiding high-sugar juices) and maintaining activity levels where possible to balance intake with needs.

A balanced diet combined with exercise is promoted to manage weight, as it helps optimize energy use and reduces risks like heart disease or pressure ulcers (Society M, 2021).

Protein: Protein is considered a key component of a balanced diet for tissue growth and repair in people with MS (Society M, 2021). Evidence indicates that high intake of animal proteins, especially red meat, may be linked to increased MS risk (t Hart, 2016), although unprocessed red meat has shown a possible protective effect in women in some studies (Black et al., 2019). In contrast, dietary intake of plant-based proteins is recommended in MS patients due to protective effects (Zielińska & Michońska, 2022). Supplementation with tryptophan in a whey protein mix has been shown to improve memory in MS patients, though no effect on mood was observed (Lieben et al., 2018). Moreover, in cases of weight loss due to symptoms like tremor or poor appetite, "food fortification" with additions such as cheese or cream is suggested to help meet nutritional needs, including protein.

Carbohydrates: Carbohydrates are a primary source of energy and play a crucial role in the diet of individuals with MS (Society M, 2021). A high-fiber diet rich in fruits, vegetables, legumes, and whole grains, while being low in simple sugars (<10% of energy, as recommended by the DGA) such as sweets and sugary drinks, has been linked to reduced disability levels (Agriculture UDoHaHSUDo, 2015; Fitzgerald et al., 2018). High-fiber carbohydrates can also help maintain a healthy gut microbiota, which may influence immune function and inflammation (Cavalla et al., 2022).

Fat: Fat intake plays a critical role in MS due to its influence on myelin integrity and inflammatory processes. SFAs, mainly from animal products, may increase circulating LDL and oxidized lipids, which are associated with adverse MS outcomes (Esparza et al., 1995; Zhornitsky et al., 2016). Low-saturated fat diets, such as the Swank diet, limit SFA from meat and dairy products to ≤15 g/day and instead emphasize mono- and polyunsaturated fatty acids (MUFA & PUFA), such as olive, safflower, sunflower, soybean, sesame, canola, flaxseed, cottonseed, linseed, and peanut oils, in amounts appropriate for energy needs (20–50 g/day), showing neuroprotective effects and potential reduction in relapse rates and disability (Foundation SM, n.d.). In addition, fish oil, through its anti-inflammatory and neuroprotective effects, may reduce nitric oxide and cytokine levels (Ramirez-Ramirez et al., 2013), and supplementation with omega-3 and fish oils has been associated with lower relapse rates, reduced inflammation, and improved QOL in MS patients (AlAmmar et al., 2021).

12.3.5 Micronutrients Requirements and Supplementations

Vitamin D: In patients with MS, having vitamin D levels below 40 ng/mL is associated with an increased risk of relapses and lesion formation (Raymond, 2023; Fitzgerald et al., 2015).

Vitamin A: Serum levels of vitamin A have been reported to be lower in patients with MS (Naziroglu et al., 2014). Retinoic acid, in combination with IFN-β1b, can enhance the restoration of impaired T-suppressor cell function (Qu et al., 1998). Moreover, vitamin A supplementation in the form of retinyl palmitate has been shown to suppress the progression of upper limb and cognitive disabilities in MS patients (Bitarafan et al., 2015). Overall, vitamin A supplementation may be beneficial in reducing inflammation and protecting the brain, particularly in patients at degenerative stages of the disease (Khosravi-Largani et al., 2018).

Vitamin E: Serum levels of vitamin E and the vitamin E/cholesterol ratio were significantly lower in patients with MS (Jiménez-Jiménez et al., 1998). Additionally, levels of alpha-tocopherol and glutathione were reduced in demyelinating plaques of MS patients (Langemann et al., 1992). Natural dietary intake of vitamin E appears to have no significant protective effect (Khosravi-Largani et al., 2018). However, increased serum concentrations of alpha-tocopherol have been associated with a reduced likelihood of simultaneous and subsequent disease activity (Løken-Amsrud et al., 2013).

Vitamin K: Studies have highlighted the significance of the vitamin K-dependent gene, Growth Arrest Specific 6 (Gas6), in the progression of MS. This gene is believed to support oligodendrocyte survival, thereby promoting myelination in the central nervous system. Additionally, Gas6 plays a key role in sphingolipid synthesis, which appears to be important for remyelination (Binder et al., 2011; Sainaghi et al., 2013; Popescu et al., 2018).

Vitamins C: The consumption of vitamin C through a regular diet does not seem to provide a meaningful protective effect. Supplementation with vitamin C, despite its antioxidant properties, may aggravate the patient's condition by triggering the Fenton reaction in the white matter of the CNS (Khosravi-Largani et al., 2018).

B Vitamins: B vitamins play key roles in cellular metabolism, nervous system function, myelin synthesis, and regulation of inflammatory pathways (Hanna et al., 2022). Deficiencies in B9 and B12 are associated with elevated homocysteine and neural damage in relapsing-remitting multiple sclerosis (RRMS) patients (Mashayekhi et al., 2024). B6 contributes to neurotransmitter and myelin synthesis (Calderón-Ospina & Nava-Mesa, 2020), B3 supports anti-inflammatory effects and lipid/DNA metabolism (Bruckert et al., 2010; Offermanns & Schwaninger, 2015), and B1 is involved in fatigue reduction and cellular activity regulation (Costantini et al., 2013). However, the role of B vitamin supplementation in preventing or improving MS symptoms remains inconclusive (Nemazannikova et al., 2018).

Minerals: Adequate intake of calcium, potassium, and other minerals has protective effects (Ghadirian et al., 1998), though direct evidence for MS outcomes is limited. Observational studies suggest that people with MS tend to have lower selenium levels compared to the general population; however, animal studies indicate that selenium supplementation may exacerbate MS-like symptoms (Raymond, 2023).

12.4 Food–Drug Interactions

While there is currently no cure for MS and no medication that directly reverses the disease, pharmacological treatments can help manage its associated symptoms, including fatigue, spasticity, tremor, pain, and mood or cognitive disturbances. Table 12.1 provides a summary of the main drug classes used in MS, their typical examples, and relevant considerations for food–drug interactions (Loleit et al., 2014; Clinic M, n.d.; Drugs.com, n.d.; Schapiro, 2002; IA A, 2014; Tavazzi et al., 2014; JL MLR, 2020; Rastkar et al., 2023; Forsah et al., 2024; Gelow, 2024; Yasaei et al., 2024; Wellness E, 2024; Clinic M, 2025a; Clinic M, 2025b; Drugs.com, 2025).

Table 12.1 Commonly prescribed medications for multiple sclerosis and their food–drug interactions

Drug	Trade name	Food–drug interactions
Immunomodulator		
Glatiramer acetate	Copaxone	**Side effects:** Hepatic, allergic, neurological, thyroid, psychological, cardiac; neoplasms, inflammatory bowel disease, viral diseases **Avoid:** Alcohol
Interferon β-1b	Betaseron, Extavia	Similar to Glatiramer acetate
Interferon β-1a	Avonex, Rebif	Similar to Glatiramer acetate
Antispasticity agents		
Tizanidine	Zanaflex	**Side effects:** Dry mouth **Avoid:** Alcohol
Baclofen	Lioresal	**Side effects:** Nausea, vomiting, diarrhea, dry mouth, headaches **Avoid:** Alcohol
Corticosteroids		
Methylprednisolone	Medrol	**Side effects:** Electrolyte disturbances, weakness, severe arthralgia, osteoporosis, pancreatitis **Avoid:** Alcohol
Stimulants		
Amantadine	Symmetrel	**Side effects:** Nausea, constipation **Avoid:** Alcohol

(cotinued)

(cotinued)

Drug	Trade name	Food–drug interactions
Modafinil	Provigil	**Side effects:** Nausea **Avoid:** Alcohol
Anticonvulsants		
Carbamazepine	Tegretol	**Side effects:** Nausea, vomiting **Avoid:** St John's wort, grapefruit/related citrus (limes, pomelo, Seville oranges), grapefruit juice, pomegranate, pomegranate juice, star fruit, alcohol
Gabapentin	Neurontin	**Side effects:** Fatigue, somnolence, dizziness, ataxia **Avoid:** Alcohol, protein
Antidepressants		
Amitriptyline *(TCA)*	Elavil	**Side effects:** Urinary retention, constipation **Avoid:** Alcohol
Sertraline (*SSRI*)	Zoloft	**Side effects:** Nausea, diarrhea, dry mouth **Avoid:** Tryptophan, alcohol, St John's wort, grapefruit juice, herbal products that have antiplatelet effects
Fluoxetine (*SSRI*)	Prozac	**Side effects:** Nausea, dry mouth **Avoid:** Tryptophan, alcohol, herbal products that have antiplatelet effects

Acknowledgments The authors confirm that the content, analysis, and conclusions of this manuscript are their own work. AI-based tools were used solely to assist in improving the clarity and correctness of the English language.

References

Agriculture UDoHaHSUDo. (2015). *2015–2020 dietary guidelines for Americans*. Skyhorse Publishing.

AlAmmar, W. A., Albeesh, F. H., Ibrahim, L. M., Algindan, Y. Y., Yamani, L. Z., & Khattab, R. Y. (2021). Effect of omega-3 fatty acids and fish oil supplementation on multiple sclerosis: A systematic review. *Nutritional Neuroscience, 24*(7), 569–579.

Altowaijri, G., Fryman, A., & Yadav, V. (2017). Dietary interventions and multiple sclerosis. *Current Neurology and Neuroscience Reports, 17*(3), 28.

Binder, M. D., Xiao, J., Kemper, D., Ma, G. Z., Murray, S. S., & Kilpatrick, T. J. (2011). Gas6 increases myelination by oligodendrocytes and its deficiency delays recovery following cuprizone-induced demyelination. *PLoS One, 6*(3), e17727.

Bitarafan, S., Saboor-Yaraghi, A., Sahraian, M. A., Nafissi, S., Togha, M., Beladi Moghadam, N., et al. (2015). Impact of vitamin a supplementation on disease progression in patients with multiple sclerosis. *Archives of Iranian Medicine, 18*(7), 435–440.

Black, L. J., Bowe, G. S., Pereira, G., Lucas, R. M., Dear, K., van der Mei, I., et al. (2019). Higher non-processed red meat consumption is associated with a reduced risk of central nervous system demyelination. *Frontiers in Neurology, 10*, 125.

Bridel, C., & Lalive, P. H. (2014). Update on multiple sclerosis treatments. *Swiss Medical Weekly, 144*, w14012.

Bronzini, M., Maglione, A., Rosso, R., Masuzzo, F., Matta, M., Meroni, R., et al. (2024). Lower multiple sclerosis severity score is associated with higher adherence to Mediterranean diet in subjects with multiple sclerosis from Northwestern Italy. *Nutrients, 16*(6), 880.

Bruckert, E., Labreuche, J., & Amarenco, P. (2010). Meta-analysis of the effect of nicotinic acid alone or in combination on cardiovascular events and atherosclerosis. *Atherosclerosis, 210*(2), 353–361.

Buscarinu, M. C., Romano, S., Mechelli, R., Pizzolato Umeton, R., Ferraldeschi, M., Fornasiero, A., et al. (2018). Intestinal permeability in relapsing-remitting multiple sclerosis. *Neurotherapeutics, 15*(1), 68–74.

Calderón-Ospina, C. A., & Nava-Mesa, M. O. (2020). B vitamins in the nervous system: Current knowledge of the biochemical modes of action and synergies of thiamine, pyridoxine, and cobalamin. *CNS Neuroscience & Therapeutics, 26*(1), 5–13.

Cavalla, P., Golzio, P., Maietta, D., Bosa, C., Pasanisi, M. B., Alteno, A., et al. (2022). Dietary habits, nutritional status and risk of a first demyelinating event: An incident case-control study in a southern European cohort. *Neurological Sciences, 43*(7), 4373–4380.

Choi, I. Y., Piccio, L., Childress, P., Bollman, B., Ghosh, A., Brandhorst, S., et al. (2016). A diet mimicking fasting promotes regeneration and reduces autoimmunity and multiple sclerosis symptoms. *Cell Reports, 15*(10), 2136–2146.

Clinic M. (2025a). *Glatiramer (subcutaneous route): Merative*. https://www.mayoclinic.org/drugs-supplements/glatiramer-subcutaneous-route/description/drg-20064045?utm_source=chatgpt.com

Clinic M. (2025b). *Amantadine (oral route): Merative*. https://www.mayoclinic.org/drugs-supplements/amantadine-oral-route/description/drg-20061695

Clinic M. (n.d.). *Glatiramer (subcutaneous route)—Description*. https://www.mayoclinic.org/drugs-supplements/glatiramer-subcutaneous-route/description/drg-20064045?utm_source=chatgpt.com

Cordain, L. (2018). *Nutritional deficiencies of ketogenic diets*. Colorado State University.

Costantini, A., Nappo, A., Pala, M. I., & Zappone, A. (2013). High dose thiamine improves fatigue in multiple sclerosis. *BML Case Reports, 2013*, bcr2013009144.

de la Rubia Ortí, J. E., Cuerda-Ballester, M., Sanchis-Sanchis, C. E., Lajara Romance, J. M., Navarro-Illana, E., & García Pardo, M. P. (2023). Exploring the impact of ketogenic diet on multiple sclerosis: Obesity, anxiety, depression, and the glutamate system. *Frontiers in Nutrition, 10*, 1227431.

Drugs.com. (2025). *Interferon beta-1a: Drugs.com*. https://www.drugs.com/food-interactions/interferon-beta-1a.html

Drugs.com. (n.d.). *Interferon beta-1b and alcohol/food interactions*. https://www.drugs.com/food-interactions/interferon-beta-1b.html?utm_source=chatgpt.com

Eckel, R. H., Jakicic, J. M., Ard, J. D., de Jesus, J. M., Houston Miller, N., Hubbard, V. S., et al. (2014). 2013 AHA/ACC guideline on lifestyle management to reduce cardiovascular risk: A report of the American College of Cardiology/American Heart Association task force on practice guidelines. *Circulation, 129*(25 Suppl 2), S76–S99.

Esparza, M. L., Sasaki, S., & Kesteloot, H. (1995). Nutrition, latitude, and multiple sclerosis mortality: An ecologic study. *American Journal of Epidemiology, 142*(7), 733–737.

Evans, E., Levasseur, V., Cross, A. H., & Piccio, L. (2019). An overview of the current state of evidence for the role of specific diets in multiple sclerosis. *Multiple Sclerosis and Related Disorders, 36*, 101393.

Fernández-Menéndez, S., Fernández-Morán, M., Fernández-Vega, I., Pérez-Álvarez, A., & Villafani-Echazú, J. (2016). Epstein-Barr virus and multiple sclerosis. From evidence to therapeutic strategies. *Journal of the Neurological Sciences, 361*, 213–219.

Filippini, G., Del Giovane, C., Vacchi, L., D'Amico, R., Di Pietrantonj, C., Beecher, D., et al. (2013). Immunomodulators and immunosuppressants for multiple sclerosis: A network meta-analysis. *Cochrane Database of Systematic Reviews, 2013*(6), Cd008933.

Fitzgerald, K. C., Munger, K. L., Köchert, K., Arnason, B. G., Comi, G., Cook, S., et al. (2015). Association of Vitamin D Levels with Multiple Sclerosis Activity and Progression in patients receiving interferon Beta-1b. *JAMA Neurology, 72*(12), 1458–1465.

Fitzgerald, K. C., Tyry, T., Salter, A., Cofield, S. S., Cutter, G., Fox, R., et al. (2018). Diet quality is associated with disability and symptom severity in multiple sclerosis. *Neurology, 90*(1), e1–e11.

Forsah, S. F., Ugwendum, D., Agbor, D. B. A., Ndema, N., Ndemazie, N. B., Tonpouwo, G. K., et al. (2024). Syncope secondary to concomitant ingestion of Tizanidine and alcohol in a patient with alcohol use disorder. *Cureus., 16*(3), e57249.

Foundation SM. (n.d.). *The Swank low-fat diet for the treatment of MS.* http://www.swankmsdiet.org/the-diet/

Gelow, R. H. R. (2024). *Modafinil and alcohol: Modafinil interactions with alcohol: The hope house.* https://www.thehopehouse.com/alcohol-abuse/related/modafinil-and-alcohol/?utm_source=chatgpt.com

Ghadirian, P., Jain, M., Ducic, S., Shatenstein, B., & Morisset, R. (1998). Nutritional factors in the aetiology of multiple sclerosis: A case-control study in Montreal. *Canada. Int J Epidemiol., 27*(5), 845–852.

Ghezzi, L., Tosti, V., Shi, L., Cantoni, C., Mikesell, R., Lancia, S., et al. (2025). Randomized controlled trial of intermittent calorie restriction in people with multiple sclerosis. *Journal of Neurology, Neurosurgery, and Psychiatry, 96*(2), 158–169.

Haki, M., Al-Biati, H. A., Al-Tameemi, Z. S., Ali, I. S., & Al-Hussaniy, H. A. (2024). Review of multiple sclerosis: Epidemiology, etiology, pathophysiology, and treatment. *Medicine (Baltimore), 103*(8), e37297.

Hanna, M., Jaqua, E., Nguyen, V., & Clay, J. (2022). Vitamins: Functions and uses in medicine. *The Permanente Journal, 26*(2), 89–97.

IA A. (2014). *Food-drug interactions and their impact on the pharmacotherapy [Diploma thesis].* University of Veterinary and Pharmaceutical Sciences Brno, Faculty of Pharmacy, Department of Human Pharmacology and Toxicology.

Irish, A. K., Erickson, C. M., Wahls, T. L., Snetselaar, L. G., & Darling, W. G. (2017). Randomized control trial evaluation of a modified Paleolithic dietary intervention in the treatment of relapsing-remitting multiple sclerosis: A pilot study. *Degener Neurol Neuromuscul Dis., 7*, 1–18.

Jiménez-Jiménez, F. J., de Bustos, F., Molina, J. A., de Andrés, C., Gasalla, T., Ortí-Pareja, M., et al. (1998). Cerebrospinal fluid levels of alpha-tocopherol in patients with multiple sclerosis. *Neuroscience Letters, 249*(1), 65–67.

JL MLR. (2020). *Krause's food & the nutrition care process* (15th ed.). Elsevier.

Katz, S. I. (2018). The role of diet in multiple sclerosis: Mechanistic connections and current evidence. *Current Nutrition Reports, 7*(3), 150–160.

Khan, G., & Hashim, M. J. (2025). Epidemiology of multiple sclerosis: Global, regional, national and sub-national-level estimates and future projections. *Journal of Epidemiology and Global Health, 15*(1), 21.

Khosravi-Largani, M., Pourvali-Talatappeh, P., Rousta, A. M., Karimi-Kivi, M., Noroozi, E., Mahjoob, A., et al. (2018). A review on potential roles of vitamins in incidence, progression, and improvement of multiple sclerosis. *eNeurologicalSci., 10*, 37–44.

Kökten, T., Hansmannel, F., Ndiaye, N. C., Heba, A. C., Quilliot, D., Dreumont, N., et al. (2021). Calorie restriction as a new treatment of inflammatory diseases. *Advances in Nutrition, 12*(4), 1558–1570.

Koukach, D., Aljumaily, M., Al-Attiyah, N., Al-Amer, R., Attia, Y., & Tayyem, R. (2025). From prevention to management: Exploring the impact of diet on multiple sclerosis. *Translational Neuroscience, 16*(1), 20250371.

Langemann, H., Kabiersch, A., & Newcombe, J. (1992). Measurement of low-molecular-weight antioxidants, uric acid, tyrosine and tryptophan in plaques and white matter from patients with multiple sclerosis. *European Neurology, 32*(5), 248–252.

Langer-Gould, A., Lucas, R. M., Xiang, A. H., Wu, J., Chen, L. H., Gonzales, E., et al. (2018). Vitamin D-binding protein polymorphisms, 25-Hydroxyvitamin D, sunshine and multiple sclerosis. *Nutrients, 10*(2), 184.

Lieben, C. K., Blokland, A., Deutz, N. E., Jansen, W., Han, G., & Hupperts, R. M. (2018). Intake of tryptophan-enriched whey protein acutely enhances recall of positive loaded words in patients with multiple sclerosis. *Clinical Nutrition, 37*(1), 321–328.

Løken-Amsrud, K. I., Myhr, K. M., Bakke, S. J., Beiske, A. G., Bjerve, K. S., Bjørnarå, B. T., et al. (2013). Alpha-tocopherol and MRI outcomes in multiple sclerosis—Association and prediction. *PLoS One, 8*(1), e54417.

Loleit, V., Biberacher, V., & Hemmer, B. (2014). Current and future therapies targeting the immune system in multiple sclerosis. *Current Pharmaceutical Biotechnology, 15*(3), 276–296.

Mashayekhi, F., Hadipour, E., Shabani, S., & Salehi, Z. (2024). Folate receptor alpha autoantibodies in the serum of patients with relapsing–remitting multiple sclerosis (RRMS). *Clinical Neurology and Neurosurgery, 237*, 108161.

Mohammadi, M., Mohammadi, A., Habibzadeh, A., Korkorian, R., Mohamadi, M., Shaygannejad, V., et al. (2024). Abnormal body mass index is associated with risk of multiple sclerosis: A systematic review and meta-analysis. *Obesity Research & Clinical Practice, 18*(5), 311–321.

Mowry, E. M., Azevedo, C. J., McCulloch, C. E., Okuda, D. T., Lincoln, R. R., Waubant, E., et al. (2018). Body mass index, but not vitamin D status, is associated with brain volume change in MS. *Neurology, 91*(24), e2256–e2264.

Naziroglu, M., Kutluhan, S., Ovey, I. S., Aykur, M., & Yurekli, V. A. (2014). Modulation of oxidative stress, apoptosis, and calcium entry in leukocytes of patients with multiple sclerosis by Hypericum perforatum. *Nutritional Neuroscience, 17*(5), 214–221.

Nemazannikova, N., Mikkelsen, K., Stojanovska, L., Blatch, G. L., & Apostolopoulos, V. (2018). Is there a link between vitamin B and multiple sclerosis? *Medicinal Chemistry, 14*(2), 170–180.

Novo, A. M., & Batista, S. (2017). Multiple sclerosis: Implications of obesity in Neuroinflammation. *Adv Neurobiol., 19*, 191–210.

Offermanns, S., & Schwaninger, M. (2015). Nutritional or pharmacological activation of HCA(2) ameliorates neuroinflammation. *Trends in Molecular Medicine, 21*(4), 245–255.

Penesová, A., Dean, Z., Kollár, B., Havranová, A., Imrich, R., Vlček, M., et al. (2018). Nutritional intervention as an essential part of multiple sclerosis treatment? *Physiological Research, 67*(4), 521–533.

Popescu, D. C., Huang, H., Singhal, N. K., Shriver, L., McDonough, J., Clements, R. J., et al. (2018). Vitamin K enhances the production of brain sulfatides during remyelination. *PLoS One, 13*(8), e0203057.

Preziosi, G., Gordon-Dixon, A., & Emmanuel, A. (2018). Neurogenic bowel dysfunction in patients with multiple sclerosis: Prevalence, impact, and management strategies. *Degener Neurol Neuromuscul Dis., 8*, 79–90.

Qu, Z. X., Dayal, A., Jensen, M. A., & Arnason, B. G. (1998). All-trans retinoic acid potentiates the ability of interferon beta-1b to augment suppressor cell function in multiple sclerosis. *Archives of Neurology, 55*(3), 315–321.

Ramirez-Ramirez, V., Macias-Islas, M. A., Ortiz, G. G., Pacheco-Moises, F., Torres-Sanchez, E. D., Sorto-Gomez, T. E., et al. (2013). Efficacy of fish oil on serum of TNF α, IL-1 β, and IL-6 oxidative stress markers in multiple sclerosis treated with interferon beta-1b. *Oxidative Medicine and Cellular Longevity, 2013*, 709493.

Rastkar, M., Ghajarzadeh, M., & Sahraian, M. A. (2023). Adverse side effects of Glatiramer acetate and interferon beta-1a in patients with multiple sclerosis: A systematic review of case reports. *Current Journal of Neurology., 22*(2), 115.

Raymond, J. L. M. K. (2023). *Krause and Manhan's food and the nutrition care process* (16th ed.). Elsevier.

Sainaghi, P. P., Collimedaglia, L., Alciato, F., Molinari, R., Sola, D., Ranza, E., et al. (2013). Growth arrest specific gene 6 protein concentration in cerebrospinal fluid correlates with relapse severity in multiple sclerosis. *Mediators of Inflammation, 2013*, 406483.

Santangelo, C., Vari, R., Scazzocchio, B., De Sanctis, P., Giovannini, C., D'Archivio, M., et al. (2018). Anti-inflammatory activity of extra virgin olive oil polyphenols: Which role in the prevention and treatment of immune-mediated inflammatory diseases? *Endocrine, Metabolic & Immune Disorders Drug Targets, 18*(1), 36–50.

Schapiro, R. T. (2002). Pharmacologic options for the management of multiple sclerosis symptoms. *Neurorehabilitation and Neural Repair, 16*(3), 223–231.

Simpson, S., Jr., van der Mei, I., Lucas, R. M., Ponsonby, A. L., Broadley, S., Blizzard, L., et al. (2018). Sun exposure across the life course significantly modulates early multiple sclerosis clinical course. *Frontiers in Neurology, 9*, 16.

Skartun, O., Smith, C. R., Laupsa-Borge, J., & Dankel, S. N. (2025). Symptoms during initiation of a ketogenic diet: A scoping review of occurrence rates, mechanisms and relief strategies. *Frontiers in Nutrition, 12*, 1538266.

Society M. (2021). *Diet and nutrition London: MS Society.* https://www.mssociety.org.uk/care-and-support/online-resources/diet-and-nutrition

Society NMS. (n.d.-a). *Disproved theories 2018.* https://www.nationalmssociety.org/What-is-MS/What-Causes-MS#section-5

Society NMS. (n.d.-b). *Smoking 2015.* https://www.nationalmssociety.org/NationalMSSociety/media/MSNationalFiles/Research/Stroup_T_Smoking_and_MS_20151110.pdf

Society NMS. (n.d.-c). *Diet & nutrition.* https://www.nationalmssociety.org/Living-Well-With-MS/Diet-Exercise-Healthy-Behaviors/Diet-Nutrition#section-0

Stoiloudis, P., Kesidou, E., Bakirtzis, C., Sintila, S. A., Konstantinidou, N., Boziki, M., et al. (2022). The role of diet and interventions on multiple sclerosis: A review. *Nutrients, 14*(6), 1150.

t Hart, B. A. (2016). Why does multiple sclerosis only affect human primates? *Multiple Sclerosis, 22*(4), 559–563.

Tafti, D., Ehsan, M., & Xixis, K. L. (2025). *Multiple sclerosis*. StatPearls. Treasure Island (FL): StatPearls Publishing Copyright © 2025, StatPearls Publishing LLC.

Tavazzi, E., Rovaris, M., & La Mantia, L. (2014). Drug therapy for multiple sclerosis. *CMAJ, 186*(11), 833–840.

Thomsen, H. L., Jessen, E. B., Passali, M., & Frederiksen, J. L. (2019). The role of gluten in multiple sclerosis: A systematic review. *Multiple Sclerosis and Related Disorders, 27*, 156–163.

Vojdani, A. (2015). Lectins, agglutinins, and their roles in autoimmune reactivities. *Alternative Therapies in Health and Medicine, 21*(Suppl 1), 46–51.

Wahls, T. L., Titcomb, T. J., Bisht, B., Eyck, P. T., Rubenstein, L. M., Carr, L. J., et al. (2021). Impact of the swank and Wahls elimination dietary interventions on fatigue and quality of life in relapsing-remitting multiple sclerosis: The WAVES randomized parallel-arm clinical trial. *Mult Scler J Exp Transl Clin., 7*(3), 20552173211035399.

Wellness E. (2024, August 26). *Drinking alcohol while on prednisone: Evoke wellness.* https://www.evokewellnessoh.com/blog/rinking-alcohol-while-on-prednisone/?utm_source=chatgpt.com

Wiseman, S. A., Tijburg, L. B., & van de Put, F. H. (2002). Olive oil phenolics protect LDL and spare vitamin E in the hamster. *Lipids, 37*(11), 1053–1057.

Yasaei, R. K. S., Patel, P., et al. (2024). *Gabapentin*. StatPearls [Internet]. Treasure Island (FL): StatPearls Publishing.

Zahoor, I., & Haq, E. (2017). Vitamin D and multiple sclerosis: An update. In I. S. Zagon & P. J. McLaughlin (Eds.), *Multiple sclerosis: Perspectives in treatment and pathogenesis*. Codon Publications Copyright: The Authors.

Zhornitsky, S., McKay, K. A., Metz, L. M., Teunissen, C. E., & Rangachari, M. (2016). Cholesterol and markers of cholesterol turnover in multiple sclerosis: Relationship with disease outcomes. *Multiple Sclerosis and Related Disorders, 5*, 53–65.

Zielińska, M., & Michońska, I. (2022). Macronutrients, vitamins and minerals in the diet of multiple sclerosis patients. *Postep Psychiatr Neurol., 31*(3), 128–137.

Chapter 13
Guillain-Barré Syndrome

Abstract

- Guillain-Barré syndrome (GBS) is an acute, immune-mediated peripheral neuropathy often triggered by infections (C. jejuni, Zika, influenza, CMV, EBV) or, rarely, vaccines or surgery. Symptoms include weakness, numbness, tingling, paralysis, and autonomic dysfunction.
- GBS affects ~100,000 people globally each year, with higher incidence in males and older adults; mortality is ~5%, and ~20% remain unable to walk independently after one year.
- Risk factors include recent infections, molecular mimicry triggering autoantibody production (e.g., against GM1, GD1 gangliosides), and underlying nutritional deficiencies.
- Nutritional management is crucial, particularly to prevent respiratory muscle loss, support immune function, and reduce complications such as pressure ulcers, electrolyte imbalances, and infections. Hypermetabolism and hypercatabolism increase energy and protein needs, often requiring early enteral feeding, texture-modified diets for dysphagia, supplemental snacks, and micronutrient supplementation (vitamins D, A, E, K, B12, iron, calcium). Malnutrition exacerbates axonal injury and slows recovery.
- Macronutrient recommendations: Energy intake of 40–45 kcal/kg/day; protein 2–2.5 g/kg/day; careful carbohydrate-to-fat ratio adjustment, especially in ventilated patients. Caloric contributions from lipid-based sedatives (e.g., propofol) should be included in total energy calculations.
- Micronutrients: Daily multivitamin-mineral supplementation is advised, with particular attention to vitamin D for immune regulation and T lymphocyte modulation. Correcting deficiencies may improve axonal recovery and overall prognosis.
- Pharmacological management targets symptom control with immunomodulators (IVIG), antipyretics (acetaminophen), corticosteroids (methylprednisolone), NSAIDs, anticonvulsants (gabapentin, carbamazepine), antidepressants (tricyclics, sertraline, citalopram, trazodone), anxiolytics (benzodiazepines), while considering side effects and food–drug interactions.

M. H. Rouhani et al., *The Healing Plate*, SpringerBriefs in Modern Perspectives on Disability Research, https://doi.org/10.1007/978-981-95-8150-4_13

Keywords Guillain-Barré syndrome (GBS) · Immune-mediated neuropathy · Nutritional management · Hypermetabolism · Dysphagia · Dysarthria · Enteral feeding · Macronutrients · Micronutrients · Food–drug interactions

13.1 Definition and Epidemiology

Guillain-Barré syndrome (GBS) is an uncommon but serious immune-mediated neuropathy that often follows an infection. It occurs due to autoimmune damage to the peripheral nerves, leading to symptoms such as numbness, tingling, and weakness, which may advance to paralysis (Nguyen & Taylor, 2025). Each year, approximately 100,000 new cases of GBS are reported worldwide. The incidence increases by about 20% with every additional decade of age, and unlike many autoimmune disorders, males are more frequently affected. The condition can be severe; despite the availability of current immunotherapies, the mortality rate remains close to 5%, and nearly 20% of patients are unable to walk independently 1 year after disease onset (Madden et al., 2024).

13.2 Etiology

GBS is a post-infectious, immune-mediated neuropathy in which cellular and humoral immune responses attack peripheral nerves (Khan et al., 2024). Molecular mimicry plays a central role, particularly after *Campylobacter jejuni* (*C. jejuni*) infections, where bacterial components resemble nerve gangliosides, triggering autoantibody production (Shahar, 2006; Yuki et al., 1993). Antibodies against gangliosides such as GM1 and GD1 contribute to demyelination and axonal injury (Rees et al., 1995).

Most cases follow an infection, including *C. jejuni*, Mycoplasma, influenza, cytomegalovirus, Epstein-Barr, and Zika virus, with up to 70% of patients reporting illness 1–6 weeks before GBS onset (Fokke et al., 2014; Raymond, 2023). *C. jejuni* is primarily transmitted to humans via contaminated food or water, most often through the consumption of raw or undercooked poultry, fish, unpasteurized milk, or water containing the bacteria (Lopes et al., 2021). In addition, *Zika* virus plays a notable role in GBS etiology. *Zika* is transmitted mainly by Aedes mosquitoes but can also be spread congenitally, sexually, or via blood (Metsky et al., 2017; Barbi et al., 2018). Infection can induce pro-inflammatory cytokines, contributing to nerve damage and the clinical manifestations of GBS (Peng et al., 2018).

Rarely, vaccinations may trigger GBS via similar immune mechanisms (Nguyen & Taylor, 2025; Haber et al., 2009). Additionally, rare triggers such as gluten sensitivity or surgical procedures have been reported (Eldar & Chapman, 2014).

13.3 Nutritional Management

Providing sufficient nutrition in patients with GBS is crucial, particularly to prevent the loss of respiratory muscles. Since adult respiratory distress syndrome is the leading cause of death in these patients and may require mechanical ventilation, proper nutritional support becomes even more important. Inadequate nutrition makes patients more vulnerable to respiratory complications due to reduced immune function, muscle wasting, and decreased respiratory muscle endurance. It also raises the risk of pressure ulcers, fluid and electrolyte imbalances, and infections (Roubenoff et al., 1992). Therefore, nutritional management in these patients is of great importance to improve neurologic functioning and overall prognosis (Escott-Stump, 2015).

13.3.1 Nutritional Challenges

Patients with GBS frequently experience hypermetabolism similar to the stress response observed in neurotrauma. Oropharyngeal muscle involvement can lead to dysphagia and dysarthria, complicating oral intake and raising the risk of aspiration (Raymond, 2023; Leonard, 2019). They commonly exhibit a hypermetabolic and hypercatabolic state driven by endocrine, infectious, and inflammatory responses, which increases their energy and protein needs (Roubenoff et al., 1992). Rapid weight loss and malnutrition, particularly hypoalbuminemia, are frequently observed in GBS induced by diet or bariatric surgery, which may exacerbate axonal injury and worsen outcomes (Wu et al., 2025). Upon hospital admission, many patients also present with additional nutritional risk factors, including dependence on mechanical ventilation, impaired gastrointestinal motility such as adynamic ileus, prior viral illnesses with gastrointestinal complications, cranial nerve deficits affecting oral intake and gut function, and reduced serum transferrin levels (Roubenoff et al., 1992). These factors, combined with the elevated metabolic demands, highlight the high nutritional vulnerability of GBS patients and the importance of early nutritional assessment and intervention.

13.3.2 General Dietary Recommendations

Nasogastric or gastric tube feeding should be initiated early and gradually to ensure adequate nutritional support. Continuous enteral feeding is generally better tolerated than bolus regimens (Meena et al., 2011). For patients with dysphagia, assessment by a speech-language pathologist is essential, and texture-modified diets may be required (Raymond, 2023). Supplemental snacks and nutrient-dense liquids may help offset unintentional weight loss (Escott-Stump, 2015). Food safety education is also important, especially regarding the prevention of *C. jejuni* infection, a common antecedent of GBS (Raymond, 2023).

13.3.3 Energy and Macronutrients Requirements

Caloric Intake: Energy expenditure in GBS patients can be markedly elevated, with indirect calorimetry indicating requirements of 40–45 kcal/kg/day (Raymond, 2023).

Protein: Protein demands are nearly double those of healthy individuals, ranging from 2.0 to 2.5 g/kg/day, in order to limit muscle catabolism and support respiratory weaning (Meena et al., 2011).

Carbohydrates and Fat: Adjusting the carbohydrate-to-fat ratio is important in ventilated patients; lowering carbohydrate intake while increasing lipid provision can reduce carbon dioxide production and facilitate weaning (Escott-Stump, 2015; Zhang et al., 2024). In addition, when sedatives such as propofol are used, the caloric contribution from its lipid emulsion, providing approximately 1.1 kcal/mL as fat, must be included in total energy calculations to prevent overfeeding (DeChicco et al., 1995).

13.3.4 Micronutrients Requirements and Supplementations

Ensuring sufficient intake of vitamins and minerals is essential to support neurological recovery and immune function. A daily multivitamin-mineral supplement may be beneficial, especially in patients with poor intake (Escott-Stump, 2015). Vitamin D deficiency is frequently seen in patients with GBS, and its role in immune regulation, particularly in modulating T lymphocyte activity, is well established (Sirufo et al., 2022). Moreover, earlier studies have indicated that acute axonal neuropathy, particularly in patients experiencing weight loss, is often linked to nutritional deficiencies (Hamel & Logigian, 2018). Malnutrition is closely associated with axonal injury, and improvements in neurological function have been observed following weight gain and targeted vitamin supplementation. Deficiencies in iron, calcium, vitamin B12, and fat-soluble vitamins (A, D, E, K) are thought to directly impair neural function, further emphasizing the critical role of adequate nutrition in preventing and mitigating axonal damage (Chamberlain et al., 2021; Lombardo et al., 2021).

13.4 Food–Drug Interactions

While there is currently no cure for GBS and no medication that directly reverses the disease, pharmacological treatments can help manage its associated symptoms, including inflammation, pain, fever, mood disturbances, and anxiety. Table 13.1

Table 13.1 Commonly prescribed medications for guillain-barré syndrome and their food–drug interactions

Drug	Trade Name	Food–Drug Interactions
Immunomodulator		
Intravenous immunoglobulin (IVIG)	Gammagard	**Side effects:** Headache, fever, chills, and fatigue **Avoid:** Alcohol
Antipyretic		
Acetaminophen	Tylenol	**Side effects:** Skin rash, hypersensitivity reactions, nephrotoxicity, hematological abnormalities **Avoid:** Alcohol
Corticosteroids		
Methylprednisolone	Medrol	**Side effects:** Electrolyte disturbances, weakness, severe arthralgia, osteoporosis, and pancreatitis **Avoid:** Alcohol
Anti-inflammatory drugs		
NSAIDs	Advil, Voltaren, Aleve	**Side effects:** Affecting the gastric mucosa, renal system, cardiovascular system, hepatic system, and hematologic system **Avoid:** Alcohol
Anticonvulsants		
Carbamazepine	Tegretol	**Side effects:** Dizziness, drowsiness, ataxia, nausea, and vomiting **Avoid:** St John's wort, grapefruit/related citrus (limes, pomelo, Seville oranges), grapefruit juice, pomegranate, pomegranate juice, star fruit, alcohol
Gabapentin	Neurontin	**Side effects:** Fatigue, somnolence, dizziness, and ataxia **Avoid:** Alcohol, protein
Antidepressants		
Amitriptyline (*TCA*)	Elavil	**Side effects:** Urinary retention, constipation, xerostomia, dizziness, headache, and somnolence **Avoid:** Alcohol
Sertraline (*SSRI*)	Zoloft	**Side effects:** Nausea, diarrhea, somnolence, tremor, and fatigue **Avoid:** Tryptophan, alcohol, St John's wort, grapefruit juice, and herbal products that have antiplatelet effects
Citalopram (*SSRI*)	Celexa	**Side effects:** Drowsiness, insomnia, dizziness, headache, diaphoresis, nausea, vomiting, xerostomia, constipation, and diarrhea **Avoid:** Tryptophan, alcohol, St John's wort, and herbal products that have antiplatelet effects
Trazodone	Desyrel	**Side effects:** Headaches, fatigue, dizziness, drowsiness, somnolence, and dry mouth **Avoid:** Alcohol, tryptophan, St John's wort, herbs that have antiplatelet Effects

(continued)

Table 13.1 (continued)

Drug	Trade Name	Food–Drug Interactions
Anxiolytics		
Alprazolam	Xanax	**Side effects:** Respiratory depression, respiratory arrest, drowsiness, confusion, headache, syncope, nausea and vomiting, diarrhea, and tremors **Avoid:** Alcohol, caffeine, herbal, and natural products that cause CNS stimulation or sedation
Diazepam	Valium	Similar to alprazolam
Lorazepam	Ativan	Similar to alprazolam
Temazepam	Restoril	Similar to alprazolam

provides a summary of the main drug classes used in GBS, their typical examples, and relevant considerations for food–drug interactions (Meena et al., 2011; Brousseau et al., 2005; IA A, 2014; Liu et al., 2015; Mahan, 2020; Kim et al., 2021; Zhang et al., 2022; Arumugham, 2023; Ghlichloo, 2023; Maan & Saadabadi, 2023; Sharbaf Shoar & Padhy, 2023; Singh, 2023; Thour, 2023; Bounds, 2024; Gerriets et al., 2024; N M, 2024; Shin, 2024; Yasaei et al., 2024; Clinic M, 2025).

Acknowledgments The authors confirm that the content, analysis, and conclusions of this manuscript are their own work. AI-based tools were used solely to assist in improving the clarity and correctness of the English language.

References

Arumugham, V. B. R. A. (2023). *Intravenous immunoglobulin (IVIG)*. StatPearls [Internet]. Treasure Island (FL): StatPearls Publishing.

Barbi, L., Coelho, A. V. C., Alencar, L. C. A., & Crovella, S. (2018). Prevalence of Guillain-Barré syndrome among Zika virus infected cases: A systematic review and meta-analysis. *The Brazilian Journal of Infectious Diseases, 22*(2), 137–141.

Bounds, C. G. P. P. (2024). *Benzodiazepines*. StatPearls [Internet]. reasure Island (FL): StatPearls Publishing.

Brousseau, K., Arciniegas, D., & Harris, S. (2005). Pharmacologic management of anxiety and affective lability during recovery from Guillain-Barré syndrome: Some preliminary observations. *Neuropsychiatric Disease and Treatment, 1*(2), 145–149.

Chamberlain, C., Terry, R., Shtayyeh, T., & Martinez, C. (2021). Recognizing postoperative nutritional complications of bariatric surgery in the primary care patient: A narrative review. *Journal of Osteopathic Medicine, 121*(1), 105–112.

Clinic M. (2025). *Immune globulin (IFAS): Mayo Clinic*. https://www.mayoclinic.org/drugs-supplements/immune-globulin-ifas-intravenous-route/description/drg-20444036

DeChicco, R., Matarese, L., Hummell, A., Speerhas, R., Seidner, D., & Steiger, E. (1995). Contribution of calories from propofol to total energy intake. *Journal of the American Dietetic Association, 95*(9), A25.

Eldar, A. H., & Chapman, J. (2014). Guillain Barré syndrome and other immune mediated neuropathies: Diagnosis and classification. *Autoimmunity Reviews, 13*(4–5), 525–530.

Escott-Stump, S. (2015). *Nutrition & diagnosis-related care* (9th ed.). Academy of Nutrition and Dietetics.

Fokke, C., van den Berg, B., Drenthen, J., Walgaard, C., van Doorn, P. A., & Jacobs, B. C. (2014). Diagnosis of Guillain-Barré syndrome and validation of Brighton criteria. *Brain, 137*(Pt 1), 33–43.

Gerriets, V. A. J., Patel, P., et al. (2024). *Acetaminophen*. StatPearls [Internet]. Treasure Island (FL): StatPearls Publishing.

Ghlichloo, I. G. V. (2023). *Nonsteroidal anti-inflammatory drugs (NSAIDs)*. StatPearls [Internet]. Treasure Island (FL): StatPearls Publishing.

Haber, P., Sejvar, J., Mikaeloff, Y., & DeStefano, F. (2009). Vaccines and Guillain-Barré syndrome. *Drug Safety, 32*(4), 309–323.

Hamel, J., & Logigian, E. L. (2018). Acute nutritional axonal neuropathy. *Muscle & Nerve, 57*(1), 33–39.

IA A. (2014). *Food-drug interactions and their impact on the pharmacotherapy*. University of Veterinary and Pharmaceutical Sciences Brno, Faculty of Pharmacy, Department of Human Pharmacology and Toxicology.

Khan, S. A., Das, P. R., Nahar, Z., & Dewan, S. M. R. (2024). An updated review on Guillain-Barré syndrome: Challenges in infection prevention and control in low- and middle-income countries. *SAGE Open Medicine, 12*, 20503121241239538.

Kim, M., Lee, E. J., & Lim, K. M. (2021). Ibuprofen increases the hepatotoxicity of ethanol through potentiating oxidative stress. *Biomol Ther (Seoul), 29*(2), 205–210.

Leonard, R. (2019). Predicting aspiration risk in patients with dysphagia: Evidence from fluoroscopy. *Laryngoscope Investig Otolaryngol, 4*(1), 83–88.

Liu, J., Wang, L. N., & McNicol, E. D. (2015). Pharmacological treatment for pain in Guillain-Barré syndrome. *Cochrane Database of Systematic Reviews, 2015*(4), CD009950.

Lombardo, M., Franchi, A., Biolcati Rinaldi, R., Rizzo, G., D'Adamo, M., Guglielmi, V., et al. (2021). Long-term iron and vitamin B12 deficiency are present after bariatric surgery, despite the widespread use of supplements. *International Journal of Environmental Research and Public Health, 18*(9), 4541.

Lopes, G. V., Ramires, T., Kleinubing, N. R., Scheik, L. K., Fiorentini, Â. M., & Padilha da Silva, W. (2021). Virulence factors of foodborne pathogen Campylobacterjejuni. *Microbial Pathogenesis, 161*(Pt A), 105265.

Maan, J. S. D. T., & Saadabadi, A. (2023). *Carbamazepine*. StatPearls [Internet]. Treasure Island (FL): StatPearls Publishing.

Madden, J., Spadaro, A., Koyfman, A., & Long, B. (2024). High risk and low prevalence diseases: Guillain-Barré syndrome. *The American Journal of Emergency Medicine., 75*, 90–97.

Mahan, L. K. R. J. (2020). *Krause's food & the nutrition care process* (15th ed.). Elsevier.

Meena, A., Khadilkar, S., & Murthy, J. (2011). Treatment guidelines for Guillain–Barré syndrome. *Annals of Indian Academy of Neurology., 14*(Suppl1), S73–S81.

Metsky, H. C., Matranga, C. B., Wohl, S., Schaffner, S. F., Freije, C. A., Winnicki, S. M., et al. (2017). Zika virus evolution and spread in the Americas. *Nature, 546*(7658), 411–415.

N M. (2024) *The dangers of drinking on prednisone: Evoke Wellness at Hilliard*. https://www.evokewellnessoh.com/blog/rinking-alcohol-while-on-prednisone/?utm_source=chatgpt.com

Nguyen, T. P., & Taylor, R. S. (2025). *Guillain-Barre syndrome*. StatPearls. Treasure Island (FL): StatPearls Publishing Copyright © 2025, StatPearls Publishing LLC.

Peng, J., Zhang, H., Liu, P., Chen, M., Xue, B., Wang, R., et al. (2018). IL-23 and IL-27 levels in serum are associated with the process and the recovery of Guillain-Barré syndrome. *Scientific Reports, 8*(1), 2824.

Raymond, J. L. M. K. (2023). *Krause and Mahan's food & the nutrition care process* (16th ed., p. 1280). Elsevier.

Rees, J. H., Gregson, N. A., & Hughes, R. A. (1995). Anti-ganglioside GM1 antibodies in Guillain-Barré syndrome and their relationship to campylobacter jejuni infection. *Annals of Neurology, 38*(5), 809–816.

Roubenoff, R. A., Borel, C. O., & Hanley, D. F. (1992). Hypermetabolism and hypercatabolism in Guillain-Barré syndrome. *JPEN Journal of Parenteral and Enteral Nutrition, 16*(5), 464–472.

Shahar, E. (2006). Current therapeutic options in severe Guillain-Barré syndrome. *Clinical Neuropharmacology, 29*(1), 45–51.

Sharbaf Shoar, N. F. K., & Padhy, R. K. (2023). *Citalopram*. StatPearls [Internet]. Treasure Island (FL): StatPearls Publishing.

Shin, J. J. S. A. (2024). *Trazodone*. StatPearls [Internet]. Treasure Island (FL): StatPearls Publishing.

Singh, H. K. S. A. (2023). *Sertraline*. StatPearls [Internet]. Treasure Island (FL): StatPearls Publishing.

Sirufo, M. M., Magnanimi, L. M., Ginaldi, L., & De Martinis, M. (2022). Guillain-Barré syndrome, the IL-33/ST2 axis, and vitamin D. *European Journal of Neurology, 29*(7), e20–e21.

Thour, A. M. R. (2023). *Amitriptyline*. StatPearls [Internet]. Treasure Island (FL): StatPearls Publishing.

Wu, Q., Li, F. Y., Hu, J., Xu, W., Feng, T. Q., Zhou, H. S., et al. (2025). Guillain-Barré syndrome following weight loss: A review of five diet-induced cases and nineteen bariatric surgery cases. *Frontiers in Neurology, 16*, 1557515.

Yasaei, R. K. S., Patel, P., et al. (2024). *Gabapentin*. StatPearls [Internet]. Treasure Island (FL): StatPearls Publishing.

Yuki, N., Taki, T., Inagaki, F., Kasama, T., Takahashi, M., Saito, K., et al. (1993). A bacterium lipopolysaccharide that elicits Guillain-Barré syndrome has a GM1 ganglioside-like structure. *The Journal of Experimental Medicine, 178*(5), 1771–1775.

Zhang, B., Duan, L., Ma, L., Cai, Q., Wu, H., Chang, L., et al. (2022). Rapidly progressive Guillain-Barré syndrome following amitriptyline overdose and severe Klebsiella pneumoniae infection: A case report and literature review. *Front Med (Lausanne), 9*, 991182.

Zhang, X., Mo, J., Yang, K., Tan, T., Zhao, C., & Qin, H. (2024). Low-carbohydrate diet score and chronic obstructive pulmonary disease: A machine learning analysis of NHANES data. *Frontiers in Nutrition, 11*, 1519782.

Index

M. H. Rouhani et al., *The Healing Plate*, SpringerBriefs in Modern Perspectives on Disability Research, https://doi.org/10.1007/978-981-95-8150-4

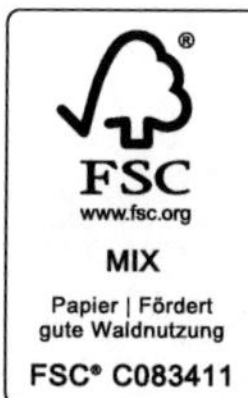

Zeitfracht Medien GmbH
Ferdinand-Jühlke-Straße 7
99095 Erfurt, Deutschland
produktsicherheit@kolibri360.de